THE GOOD HOUSEWIFE'S JEWEL

THE GOOD HOUSEWIFE'S JEWEL

By

THOMAS DAWSON

With an introduction by Maggie Black

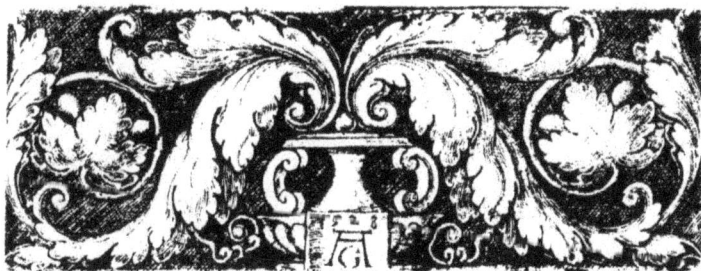

eǫuinox

SHEFFIELD UK   BRISTOL CT

Published by Equinox Publishing Ltd

UK: Office 415, The Workstation, 15 Paternoster Row, Sheffield, South Yorkshire S1 2BX

USA: ISD, 70 Enterprise Drive, Bristol, CT 06010

www.equinoxpub.com

First published by Southover Press 1996
This edition published by Equinox Publishing 2018

© Introduction Maggie Black 1996

British Library Cataloguing-in-Publication Data

A catalogue record for this book is available from the British Library

ISBN-13   978 1 87096 212 4 (hardback)
          978 1 78179 851 5 (ePDF)

Printed and bound by Lightning Source Inc. (La Vergne, TN), Lightning Source UK Ltd. (Milton Keynes), Lightning Source AU Pty. (Scoresby, Victoria).

CONTENTS

INTRODUCTION

Thomas Dawson wrote or, possibly, compiled the cookery book now in front of me in 1596 and 1597 when English society stood on the threshold of a new era. Although profiteering and inflation had reduced thousands of the poor and spendthrift to a sad plight or even to vagrancy, traders, especially in the towns, were making profits, and there were other signs of economic turn round. Compared with the rural poor, city artisans lived quite well in Elizabethan England, and so did landowners shrewd enough to dabble in commerce or the gamble of overseas investment. Merchants and middling professional men did even better, and were more or less indistinguishable from gentlemen in style, dress, and habits.

It is interesting , for instance, to see how a London citizen entertained friends to dinner informally at home as Claudius Hollyband, a French immigrant teacher, described it in the school books he wrote for his pupils while living at Lewisham in the 1570s. Hollyband, who had anglicised his name, chose the device of dialogues or playlets to list the French terms he wanted his pupils to learn; although sometimes, for example in Lesson 4 called *School Meals*, when the boys asked a guest to supper before 'prep', the arrangements were somewhat haphazard, and the number of dishes was certainly larger than any schoolboy would normally get, in order to cover as many synonyms as possible.

It will not take any modern reader long to realise that this pleasantly relaxed teacher laced his lessons well with praises to encourage his pupils. Nonetheless, they are of more interest to us for the descriptions they give of typical everyday meals enjoyed by normal, healthy Elizabethans, young and old, and the people who served them. We are told their mealtimes — breakfast at seven, dinner at eleven or near it, supper at five. We note that even the rather testy host expects to dish out hospitality freely, at least on Sundays, and trusts his more careful servants to broach his wine and serve it. However he expects his Sunday guests, who are usually cousins or other near relatives, to sit where he bids them after washing their hands, and he insists that his children say grace before and after the meal when they are at home. This Elizabethan citizen gives care and time to his children's welfare as well as their discipline, or so Hollybrand alleges (but then he would say that, wouldn't he?). The youngsters have been allocated two servants to see to their needs. The senior servant, perhaps thinking himself worthy of better status, takes his annoyance out on his saucy junior, accusing him of tasting the dishes in the kitchen, and helping himself to the gravy and sausages, and perhaps other titbits.

While this is going on, the grownups' meal is laid, and our citizen and his nearest cousin exchange teasing comments about the wine. Powdered (salted) beef and mustard was a standard 'starter' in Elizabethan times and it is served by our citizen with a suitably derisory comment on his cousin's rubicund complexion, while the junior serving-boy, William, who always seems to be in trouble, is told to complete the table arrangement and give porridge and spoons to the children at the same time. Soon it is little John's turn to be scolded — and then the master of the house starts complaining about some over-spiced cabbages, and mutton stuffed with garlic; he would have preferred some capon boiled with leeks before the second course, including the roasts, is served. This course, when it comes, consists of larded shoulder of veal, cold turkey and chicken, with a particularly good claret to drink, and also a venison pasty (always a favourite), blackbirds, larks, and woodcocks, partridge and a roast hare wih 'black' (blood thickened) sauce.

The unexpected arrival of litle John's godparents creates a stir, but any unease is overcome by the fact that they have come from seeing the Queen give an audience to an aged dame. The dessert is then served to most of the guests while the newcomers —— are they perhaps catholics? — are offered fish (dressed carp and pike) before joining the others. They all then consume baked pears with scraped cheese, pippins, tarts, custard pies and cake, roasted chestnuts, and a choice of cheeses ranging from French angelot to parmesan and gouda. When that has been eaten, young Henry says grace, and everyone gets ready to go the second Church service of the day.

We tend to think of the Elizabethans as robust in health and able to take on most of the hazards encountered in everyday life. It is all too easy to overlook the deaths of the new-born, teenagers struck down by smallpox, mothers in labour, and the middle-aged killed slowly and painfully by kidney or bladder stones. Thomas Dawson did not, himself, attempt to cope with most such disasters in his recipe book; more sensibly he dealt with first aid and tummy upsets. But he did give a recipe for alleviating, if not curing, the dreaded stone, and made a valuable connecton between diet and health-giving herbs, which are now so much more accurately recognised than they were then, and are increasingly accept- able as cures or at least palliatives.

Thomas Dawson's background is not otherwise very clear to us. He may have been a great man's gardener, just as John Gerard was Lord Burghley's, or may have been a steward or master cook. Anyway, he certainly had access to a fairly big herb garden and probably to a spice merchant's or apoth- ecary's shop where he could obtain exotic fresh as well as dried fruits and vegetables. We know this because his book tells us that he was the first person to publish a recipe for sweet potatoes some months at least before Gerard's Herball was printed. It is quite therefore possible that the two men were colleagues, if not cronies, and may well have had some training in herbal medicine together as part of their chosen studies. It seems likely, at any rate, that most of his knowledge of animal husbandry was acquired in England, possibly some of it from early versions of Gervase Markham's treatises such as *The English Hus-wife*; plagiarism was not a sin in those days, and Markham himself used his writings more than once, with long intervals between. Dawson certainly focussed more on meat and poultry dishes than anything else. It is noticeable that he only gave one recipe for a cheese dish, one omelet, and very few fricasees, although he did offer some sweet dishes such as trifle and a cast (clotted) cream dish. The sauces with which Dawson garnished his dishes were old-fashioned ones, such as green (parsley) sauce and black sauce. He also offered a white broth with almonds, and other 'fysshe daye' fare which he may have picked up from a much older book or manuscript.

He seems to have been a tidy-minded fellow, as befitted a gardener or cook. With very few exceptions, his recipes and notes are clearly the work of a man who, though naive at times compared with some Court contemporaries, went straight to the point of what he had to say without wasting time on long words. Take, for instance, the section of his book that deals with 'boyled' (we would say 'poached') small birds, rabbits, and water fowl, followed by similar recipes for larger birds and meats, then offal and pies. No wastage here! I must grant that in many of his recipes the subjects are diverse, and sometimes unusual, perhaps just for the sake of diversity. But they are none the worse for that because Dawson did not elaborate, it seems to me, just to show off, but more likely in order to note something which had only just occurred to him, or to nurture some plant which he had been hoping to find a place for because he liked its scent or shape.

This stands out noticably in the material which he has gathered together to describe his medical receipts (mostly derived from medieval manuscripts). Probably none of us, even the most avid historians, will want to experiment with the first medicament on page,which is a mixture of orpiment (arsenic trisulphide) and verdigris, ground up and bagged for keeping (is this a forerunner of Kenelm Digby's ploys?).

Luckily the recipes which follow only appear to be quaint and not dangerous, and Dawson's 'Approved points of Husbandrie' are a true countryman's way of dealing with livestock, whether intended for field work or for the table. They remind me of the emphasis he laid on using 'fair', that is, clear water in both his recipes and his drinks. His herbal cures almost all sound pleasantly simple to use too. Fennel, parsley, alexanders, borage, pennyroyal, violet leaves, cinquefoil, succory, endive, hollyhock leaves, mallow leaves, red garden mint, dandelion roots and liquorice provide just one batch of ingredients; their seeds and those of coriander and cumin being added in the boiling. Two recipes for imperial water to cure wounds and fungal infections are given, and two for distilled cinnamon water, then two flower distillates and three 'hopeful' recipes to ease the pain of the stone. The last group of recipes are for plasters to apply to shingles or to cramped, shortened or torn sinews, and some extras for staunching blood, shrinking swellings, for slimming (dear me!) and for soothing scabs and itching. Lastly, despite the calm of the Queen's last years, Dawson supplied an antidote for poison and a recipe to cure anyone struck speechless.

In the later part of his book, Dawson reverted to cookery and to dishes for discriminating families interested in new ideas. Now we see him as an artist at work, producing meals in which the majority of dishes contained one item , at least, produced with real flair, using quite simple ingredients but very carefully chosen. Mutton or veal with mock pears, stuffed cabbage, a pot pie and a mock venison pâte in a crust are among many good examples, followed by an all-purpose herb and fruit stuffing which I can vouch for.

Dawson must, I think, have had some aristoratic client or employer, to judge by the galantine on page 114, his big and little pies and cream tarts, and jelly decorated with gold leaf. Perhaps continental contacts too, if we accept his use of a 'dish of butter' as a meatless starter, his instrucions for cooking carp, succeeded by pike with oranges, and other fish such as conger and fresh salmon. No one would want to try porpoise steaks today. In general however, it is interesting to compare Dawson's dishes with the more wide-ranging recipes produced by Gervase Markham in his major works. No English cook worth his salt would forget his drink, Dawson certainly does not. Do his surrealist-sounding boiled pig's feet with bastard not appeal? Try calling them Trotters with rich wine and cook them in brown sherry with a touch of vinegar and honey. Or try Andrew Boorde's spiced, slightly sharp, respyse (raspberry-flavoured) wine or the better known hypocras. Elizabethan and Stuart diners went overboard for such piments, as these concocted drinks were called.

One's questionings are further aroused by Dawson's delightful (for me) collection of salad recipes which, with some adaptations (I shall skip the periwinkles and whelks) will cheer up my own less appealing starters. I will go further and say that Dawson's salmon and trout recipes are the best historical fish recipes I have seen for some time.

After a few egg dishes, Dawson turned his talents to preserves, in perhaps the book's most charming section to read, if not to make, because candying is a notoriously laborious task. It is difficult however, *not* to be beguiled by the prospect of preserved cherries, candied green walnuts, and musk-flavoured melons, or pickled vine fruits. Search, too, for the spice-stuffed rolled veal slices (aloes) and follow them with a citron pie. For a New Year celebration dish, try one of Dawson's recipes for haggis, or his stuffed roast pig, or roast hare with stiff peach conserve. Such accompaniments are not as strange as you may think, and can be surprisingly good.

Whenever I think of Thomas Dawson, his unknown pedigree and now lost experience, (he was obviously a practised if not a professional cook) I cannot help comparing his crisp common-sense with the more laborious work of scholars in his own generation and the Court cooks in the next. He emerges from the text very much his own man, belonging to neither group. By birth he was clearly an Elizabethan, and perhaps Shakespeare's near contemporary, born in the 1560s or 70s, and he seems to have travelled, at least in France because he mentions French animal husbandry as if he knows it at first hand. But even of that we cannot be quite sure, because he may well have been only the compiler of this book which bears his name. There are significant discrepancies between the spellings in the earlier and later material which point to that possibility although not conclusively; and some repetitions suggest that another writer may have contributed alternative versions or repeats of certain recipes, which for some reason Dawson kept in his text. As I've said, the whole work was published in two parts, in 1596 and 1597 and that is all we can claim with certainty. Yet does it matter very much whose hand actually held the quill which penned these recipes? Does it even matter if it was one hand or several? I rather think not. Surely what matters most is the accuracy of the content and the style. If these are consistent, competent and a pleasure to read and to use, all the way through the book, we should have no concern.

There is just one snag. In my experience, there is no such thing as a perfect cookery manuscript or even a perfect recipe. However strictly one disciplines one's ideas, possible variations, if not faults, creep into the tidiest text or grammatical structure, and in the end, the reader not the writer must choose what to do with his material, and how to phrase it, because its vitality will depend on his or her input. Thomas Dawson's text is easier to deal with than those of his contemporaries and most of his successors because it is simpler. As far as there can be an Elizabethan cookery book without fault, Thomas Dawson and his modern scribe have created it. I hope it will give you as much pleasure as it has given me.

MAGGIE BLACK

SOURCES

A Leech Book or Collection of Medical Recipes of the 15th century. The text of the Medical Society of London together with a transcript. Ed. Warren R Dawson. Macmillan and Co Ltd 1934.

An Ordinance of Pottage. An edition of the 15th century culinary receipts in Yale University's MS Beinnecke 163. With a commentary on the recipes by Constance B Hieatt. Prospect Books 1988.

The Elizabethan Home discovered in two dialogues by Claudius Hollyband and Peter Erondell. Ed. M St Clair Byrne. Methuen and Co 1949.

Burton, Elizabeth. *The Elizabethans at Home.* Longmans Group Ltd. 1958.

Younger, William. *Gods, Men and Wine.* Michael Joseph for the Wine and Food Society. 1966.

Drummond, Jack, and Wilbraham, Anne. *The Englishman's Food.* Jonathan Cape. 1969.

EDITOR'S NOTE

Thomas Dawson's book was published in two parts, one part in 1596 and the other a year later. The recipes in it are all jumbled together throughout both parts, and several are in duplicate. In order to make it easier to cook from I have put the different methods of cooking together, using very broad headings. Boiling is the largest section. It was, of course, easier to poach over a fire than roast in front of one or bake in an oven, given the rather primitive equipment then in use. The baking section is nearly all concerned with meat and fruit cooked in pastry (coffins), or open tarts.

The collection stands midway between medieval cookery and the beginning of a more modern style at the end of the seventeenth century. Two very interesting echoes of the medieval tradition appear in it, sandwiched between recipes for every day. The first is the ornate centrepiece of a stuffed, that is farced, bird or animal — in Dawson's case a pullet stuffed and dressed as a two-headed spread eagle. The second is the list and recipes for Banqueting Stuff, the highly decorated course so loved by the Elizabethans, that followed a full dinner, made of marchpane (marzipan) in different shapes and colours, and some ideas for fashioning it into fruit, cups, glasses, and plates. Several recipes give directions for colouring food, from saunders blue and egg yolk and saffron, to gold leaf, added when the dish was complete, and instructions for preparing the gold for use. The gold leaf, saffron yellow, azurite blue, green from spinach, and the very white dishes made from curds, together with green, white, and black sauces must have made a varied and colourful design on the table.

Nearly all the recipes are cookable now. The ubiquitous seasoning of cinnamon and ginger, if used rather sparingly, is a delicious addition and deserves to be revived. In fact, this is a useful source book of tastes and ideas.

Although quantities are rather vague, a handful of this or that, when a pint measure is given it is essential to remember that at this time, predating the imperial pint, the measure is 16 fluid ounces instead of 20.

Only the erratic punctuation has been altered and an excessive use of the word 'and' has been reduced. Where I have added a word it appears in square brackets in the text. The first time an unusual word or ingredient is used in a recipe there is a note with an asterisk. The term also appears in the glossary. The best reason for resetting the text in a modern typeface is that it is easier to read. A facsimile page of the original appears at the end of the book.

I am much indebted to Tessa McKirdy and Ann Morgan Hughes, to Uta Schumacher-Voelker for her kindness and help with the words in the recipes that defeated us, and to both Nicholas and Catharine Bagnall, without whose unstinting work I doubt whether this edition would have ever been completed.

A.B.

SOURCES OF ILLUSTRATIONS

Robert May, *The Accomplisht Cook:* Hannah Woolley, *The Queen-like Closet or Rich Cabinet:* Ibn-Butlan, *Elimithar Elluchasem:* T. Hall, *The Queen's Royal Cookery:* Buffon, *Natural History:* B. Scappi, *Opera dell'Arte Cucinare:* and *Opera di M. Barrtolemeo Scappi Cuoco Secreto di Papa Pio V.* Lobera de Avila, *Banket der Hofe imd Edenent:* N. Culpeper, *Complete Herbal:* Heindrich Aldegrever, Engraving.

THE
good huſvvifes
Iewell.

VVherein is to be found moſt excel-
lend and rare Deuiſes for conceites in
Cookery, found out by the prac-
tiſe of Thomas Dawſon.

Wherevnto is adioyned ſundry approued
receits for many ſoueraine oyles, and
the way to diſtill many precious
waters, with diuers approued
medicines for many
diſeaſes.

*Alſo certain approued points of huſbandry, very
neceſſary for all Husbandmen to know.*

Newly ſet foorth with additions. 1596.

Imprinted at London for *Edward White,*
dwelling at the litle North doore of
Paules at the ſigne of the Gun.

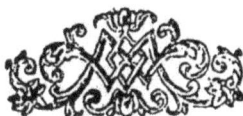

Here followeth the order of meats, how they must be served at the table with their sauces for flesh days at dinner.

THE FIRST COURSE

Potage or stewed broth. Boiled meat or stewed meat. Chickens and Bacon. Powdered Beef. Pies. Goose. Pig. Roasted Beef. Roasted Veal. Custard.

THE SECOND COURSE

Roasted Lamb. Roasted Capons. Roasted Conies. Chickens. Peahens. Baked Venison. Tart.

THE FIRST COURSE AT SUPPER

A salad. A Pig's pettitoe. Powdered Beef, sliced. A shoulder of Mutton or a breast. Veal. Lamb. Custard.

THE SECOND COURSE

Capons roasted. Conies roasted. Chickens roasted. Pigeons roasted. Larks roasted. A pie of Pigeons or Chickens. Baked Venison. Tart.

THE SERVICE AT DINNER

A dozen Quails. A dish of Larks. Two pasties of Red Deer in a dish. Tart. Gingerbread. Fritters.

SERVICE FOR FISH DAYS

Butter. A salad with hard Eggs. Potage of Sand Eels and
Lampreys. Red Herring green broiled, strewed upon. White
Herring. Ling. Haburdine:* sauce, mustard. Salt Salmon,
minced. Two pasties of Fallow Deer in a dish. A Custard. A
dish of Leeches.
* *A large cod now mostly used for salting.*

THE SECOND COURSE

Jelly. Peacocks: sauce, wine and salt. Two Conies or half a
dozen Rabbits: sauce, mustard and sugar. Half a dozen of
Pigeons. Mallard. Zoyle:* sauce, mustard and verjuice. Gulls.
Stork. Herons. Crab: sauce, galantine. Curlew. Bittern. Bustard.
Pheasant: sauce, water and salt with onions sliced. Half a
dozen Woodcocks: sauce, mustard and sugar. Half a dozen
Teals: sauced as the Pheasants. A dozen of Quails. A dish of
Larks. Two pasties of Red Deer in a dish. Tart. Gingerbread.
Fritters.
* *Sole.*

SERVICE FOR FISH DAYS

Butter. A salad with hard Eggs. Potage of Sand Eels and
Lampreys. Red Herring, green broiled, strewed upon. White
Herring. Ling. Harburdine: sauce, mustard. Salt Salmon,
minced: sauce, mustard and verjuice and a little sugar.
Powdered Conger. Shad. Mackerel: sauce, vinegar. Whiting:
sauce with the liver and mustard. Plaice: sauce, sorrel or
wine, and salt or mustard, or verjuice. Thornback: sauce,
liver and mustard, pepper and salt strewed upon after it is
bruised. Fresh Cod: sauce, green sauce. Dace. Mullet. Eels

4

upon sops. Roach upon sops. Perch. Pike in pike sauce. Trout upon sops. Tench in jelly or gorebill.* Custard.
* *Garfish.*

THE SECOND COURSE

Flounders or flokes:* pike sauce. Fresh Salmon. Fresh Conger. Brette.** Turbot. Halibut: sauce, vinager. Bream upon sops. Carp upon sops. Soles, or any other fishes, fried. Roasted Eel: sauce, the dripping. Roasted Lampreys. Roasted Porpoise. Fresh Sturgeon: sauce, galantine. Crayfish. Crab. Shrimps: sauce, vineger. Baked Lamprey. Tart. Cheese. Raisins. Pears.
* *Ling.*
** *A species of turbot.*

FINIS

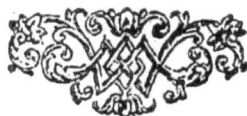

BOILING

STEWING

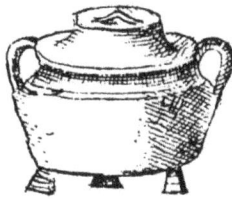

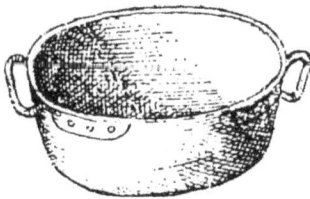

TO BOIL LARKS

Take sweet bread and strain it into a pipkin and set it on the fire. And put in a piece of butter and skim it as clean as you can. Put in spinach and endive and cut it a little. And so let it boil. Put in pepper, cloves and mace, cinnamon and ginger and a little verjuice. And when you serve them up lay sops in the dish.

TO BOIL CONIES*

Take a coney and parboil it a little. Then take a good handful of parsley, and a few sweet herbs and the yolks of four hard eggs. Chop them all together, then put in pepper and a few currants and fill the conie's belly full of butter. Then prick her head between her hinder legs, and break her not. Put her into a fair earthen pot with mutton broth and the rest of the stuff. Roll it up round and put it in withal. And so boil them well together and serve it with sops.
* *Adult rabbits.*

TO BOIL A CONEY

You must boil your conie and strain your sweet bread into a pipkin and put in your meat. Skim it as clean as you can and put in a good deal of endive and cut it a little. And a good piece of butter and all kinds of spices and a little verjuice. And so serve it upon sops.

TO BOIL CHICKENS

First you shall take chickens and boil them with grapes and with a rack of mutton together. Let the rack of mutton boil before the chickens one hour and a half. Then make a bunch of herbs with rosemary, thyme, savory and hyssop

and also marjoram. Bind them fast together. Put them in the pot and when you see your time put in your chickens with parsley in their bellies and a little sweet butter*, verjuice and pepper. When you have so done, boil your grapes in a little pipkin by themselves with some of the broth of the chickens. But take heed not to boil them too much nor yet too little. Then take the yolks of five eggs and strain them with a little broth of the pot, and when they are strained put them in the pipkin to the grapes and stir them. When they begin to boil take them from the fire and stir them a good while after you have taken them up. Then have your sippets ready in a platter and lay your meat upon it. And take your pipkins and grapes and all that is in them and pour it upon the meat. And after this sort serve it in.
Unsalted butter.

TO BOIL MUTTON AND CHICKENS

Take your mutton and chickens and set upon the fire with fair water. When it is well skimmed take two handfuls of cabbage, lettuce, a handful of currants, a good piece of butter, the juice of two or three lemons, a good deal of gross pepper and a good piece of sugar. Let them seethe all well together. Then take three or four yolks of eggs together hard roasted, and strain them with part of your broth. Let them seethe a quantity of an hour. Serve your broth with meat upon sippets.

TO BOIL CHICKENS

Strain your broth into a pipkin and put in your chickens and skim them as clean as you can. Put in a piece of butter and a good deal of sorrel. And so let them boil. Put in all manner of spices and a little verjuice. Pick a few barberries, and cut a lemon in pieces, and scrape a little sugar upon them. Lay them on the chickens when you serve them up. Lay sops upon the dish.

ANOTHER WAY TO BOIL CHICKENS

You must strain your broth into a pipkin and set it aboiling and skim it. Put in a piece of butter and endive and so let it boil. And a few currants, and all manner of spices. Serve it on sops.

TO BOIL PLOVERS

You must strain your sweet broth into a pipkin and set them on the fire. And when they boil you must scum them. Then put in a piece of butter and a good deal of spinach and a little parsley, a piece of carrot cut very small, and a few currants.

And so let them boil. And all manner of spices and a little white wine, and a little verjuice, and so serve them upon sops.

TO BOIL TEALS

Take sweet broth and onions and shred them, and spinach, and put in butter and pepper. Then leave it with toasts of bread, with a little verjuice. And so serve it on sops.

TO BOIL STEAKS BETWEEN TWO DISHES

You must put parsley and currants, butter and verjuice, two or three yolks of eggs and pepper, cloves and mace, and so let them boil together. Serve them upon sops.

TO BOIL A NEAT'S TONGUE

In primis, in fair water and salt, then peel it and cut it in the middle. Then boil it in red wine and fill him full of cloves and a little sugar. Then wash it with a little sweet broth to do away the scent of the wine. You must make a little sweet muscat with red wine and prunes boiled together. Then strain it and strain a little mustard in a fine cloth together. And so serve it.

TO BOIL A CAPON

Put the capon into the ponder* beef pot, and when you think it almost tender take a little pot and put therein half water and half wine, marrow, currants, dates, whole mace, verjuice, pepper and a little thyme.
* *Heavy.*

THE BOILING OF A CAPON

Seethe the capon itself in water and salt and nothing else. To make the broth viz:
Take strong broth made with beef or mutton broth, so that it be strong broth, and put into it rosemary, parsley and thyme, and four leaves of sage. This let seethe in it a good while. Then put into it small raisins and a few whole mace. A quarter of an hour before it be ready to be taken from the fire have ready sodden* four or five eggs boiled hard. Take nothing out but the yolks. Strain the eggs with a little of the same broth and verjuice. Have a little marrow cut in small pieces and an apple pared and cut in small pieces. If that time so serve, take the best of lettuce, cutting off the tops to the white and best, and take a few prunes with two or three dates. Thus let it seethe a quarter of an hour or more.
* *Soaked.*

When it is ready to take up have your dish with sops ready and the water well strained out of the capon. Then season the broth with a little pepper. Then take it and dish it and scrape upon it a little sugar, laying the prunes round about the dish side.

TO BOIL A CAPON WITH ORANGES
AND LEMONS

Take oranges or lemons peeled, and cut them the long way. If you can keep your cloves whole put them into your best broth of mutton or capon, with prunes or currants and three or four dates. When these have been well sodden put whole pepper, great mace, a good piece of sugar, some rose water and either white or claret wine. And let all these seethe together a while. And so serve it upon sops with your capon.

TO BOIL A CAPON IN WHITE BROTH
WITH ALMONDS

Take your capon with marrow bones and set them on the fire, and when they be clean skimmed take the fattest of the broth put it in a little pot with a good deal of marrow, prunes, raisins, dates, whole maces and a pint of white wine. Then blanch your almonds and strain them. With them thicken your pot and let it seethe a good while. When it is enough serve it upon sops with your capon.

TO BOIL A CAPON IN WHITE BROTH

Take a good capon and scald him and when he is fair washed put him in your pot. Take a good marrow bone too, or, if you have no marrow bone take a neck of mutton. When your capon is half boiled take a pottle* of the

13

uppermost of your broth and put it into a fair posnet.** Then take two handfuls of fine currants and big dates, cut every one in four pieces, and four or five whole mace, four spoonfuls of verjuice, and so much sugar as an egg, a little thyme and a little parsley, a little marjoram, and if you have no marjoram then one small twig of rosemary. Bind all your herbs fast together. When you have clean washed them, put to the said herbs sugar, currants, mace, and verjuice into your posnet, and a grated nutmeg. Let them boil together and when it is almost enough, have a small handful of almonds blanched and beaten and strained with a little of the same liquor. Put that into your broth a good quarter of an hour before you take it up. That will make it white. You must also put in some good pieces of marrow, and let not the marrow and dates seethe above half an hour. You must take a good handful of prunes and tie them in clean cloths and seethe them in the broth where the capon is. When you take up your capon to serve it in, lay a few sippets in the bottom of your platter. And lay a few prunes and barberries both about the rim of the platter and upon the capon. You may boil chickens in the like sort.

* *A liquid measure of about half a gallon.*
** *A small metal pot with a handle and three legs.*

TO MAKE BOILED MEATS FOR DINNER

Take the ribs of a neck of mutton and stuff it with marjoram, savory, thyme and parsley chopped small, and currants, with the yolks of two eggs, pepper and salt. Then put it into a posnet with fair water, or else with the liquor of some meat, with vinegar, pepper and salt, and a little butter to serve it.

TO BOIL MEATS FOR SUPPER

Take veal and put it into a posnet with carrot roots cut in

long pieces. Then boil it and put thereto a handful of prunes and crumbs of bread. Then season it with pepper, salt and vinegar.

TO BOIL A LEG OF MUTTON WITH
A PUDDING

First, with a knife raise the skin round about till you come to the joints. When you have parboiled the meat, shred it fine with suet or marrow, parsley, marjoram and pennyroyal. Then season it with pepper and salt, cloves, mace and cinnamon. Then take the yolks of two or three eggs and mingle with your meat a good handful of currants and a few minced dates. Put the meat into the skin of the leg and close it with pricks. And so boil it with the broth that you boil the Capon. And let it seethe the space of two hours.

TO BOIL PIG'S FEET AND PETTITOES

Take and boil them in a pint of verjuice and bastard.* Take four dates minced with a few raisins, then take a little thyme and chop it small. Season it with a little cinnamon and ginger and a quantity of verjuice.
* *A sweet white wine.*

TO BOIL A LAMB'S HEAD AND PURTENANCE*

Strain your broth into a pipkin and set it on the fire. Put in butter and skim it as clean as you can. Put in your meat and put in endive and cut it a little. And strain a little yeast and put into it, and currants and prunes. Put in all manner of spices and so serve it upon sops.
* *Innards.*

TO BOIL QUAILS

First put them into a pot with sweet broth and set them on the fire. Then take a carrot root and cut him in pieces and put into the pot. Then take parsley and sweet herbs, and chop them a little and put them into the pot. Then take cinnamon, ginger, nutmegs and pepper, and put in a little verjuice, and so season it with salt. Serve them upon sops and garnish them with fruit.

TO BOIL PIGEONS IN BLACK BROTH

First roast them a little, then put them into an earthen pot, with a little quantity of sweet broth. Then take onions, and slice them, and set them on the coals with some butter to take away the scent of them. Put them into the pigeons, and lace it with a toast of bread drawn with vinegar. Then put some sweet herbs half cut, and cinnamon and ginger, and gross pepper, and let them boil. Season them with salt, serve them upon sops, and garnish them with fruit.

TO BOIL A MALLARD WITH CABBAGE

Take some cabbage and prick and wash them clean, and parboil them in fair water. Then put them into a collander and let water run from them clean. Then put them into a fair earthen pot, and as much sweet broth as will cover the cabbage, and sweet butter. Then take your mallard and roast it half enough, and save the dripping of him. Then cut him in the side and put the mallard into the cabbage and put in all your dripping. Let it stew an hour. Season it with salt and serve it upon sops.

TO BOIL A DUCK WITH TURNIPS

Take her first and put her into a pot with stewed broth. Then take parsley and sweet herbs and chop them and parboil the roots very well in another pot. Then put unto them sweet butter, cinnamon, ginger, gross pepper and whole mace. Season it with salt. Serve it upon sops.

TO BOIL PIE MEAT

Take a leg of mutton and mince it very fine with suet. Seethe it in a little pan or an earthen pot with butter. And season it with cloves, mace, great raisins, prunes and salt, and serve it in a dish. And if you will, put in some juice of oranges and lay half an orange upon it.

THE ORDER TO BOIL A BRAWN*

Take your brawn, and when you have cut him out lay him in fair water four and twenty hours. Shift it four or five times. Scrape and bind up those [pieces] that you think good with hemp. Bind one handful of green willows together, and lay them in the bottom of the pan. Then put in your brawn and skim it very clean. Let it boil but softly; it must be so tender that you may put a straw through it. When it is boiled enough, let it stand and roll in the pan. When you take it up let it lie in trays one hour or two. Then make [a] sousing drink with ale and water and salt; you must make it very strong. And so let it lie a week before you spend it.
* *Lean pig meat, ham or gammon.*

TO BOIL A CAPON WITH A SYRUP

Boil your capon in sweet broth, and put in gross pepper and whole mace into the capon's belly. Make your syrup with spinach, white wine, currants, sugar, cinnamon and ginger, and sweet butter. And so let them boil. When your capon is ready to serve put the syrup on the capon, and boil your spinach before you make your syrup.

TO BOIL MARROW BONES FOR DINNER

First put your marrow bones into a fair pot of water, and let them boil till they be half enough. Then take out all your broth, saving so much as will cover your marrow bones. Then put thereto eight or nine carrot roots, and see they be well scraped and washed, and cut inch long or little less, and a handful of parsley and hyssop chopped small. Season with salt, pepper and saffron. You may boil chines and racks of veal in all points as this.

TO BOIL A CAPON

Let your capon be fair scalded and short trussed, and put into a pot of water with a marrow bone or two, and a rack of mutton cut together in three or four pieces. Let them boil together till they be half boiled, then take out a ladleful or two of the best of the broth, and put it into a fair earthen pot Put thereto a pint of white wine or claret, and cut twelve or fourteen dates long ways, and a handful of small raisins, a handful of thyme, rosemary and hyssop bound together, and so let these parcels boil by themselves. When your capon is enough, lay it in a fair platter upon sops of white bread, and your mutton by him also. Then take out the marrow from the bones, whole, and lay it upon the capon and mutton. And so serve it forth. Your latter broth must be seasoned with cinnamon, cloves, and mace, and salt and mace beaten also.

TO BOIL A CAPON WITH ORANGES

Take your capon and set him on the fire as before with marrow bones and mutton, and when you have skimmed the pot well, put thereto the value of a farthing loaf, and let it boil till it be half boiled. Then take two or three ladlefuls of the same broth and put it into an earthen pot, with a pint of the wine aforesaid. Peel six or eight oranges and slice them thin, and put them into the same broth with four pennyworth in sugar or more, and a handful of parsley, thyme and rosemary, together tied. Season it with whole mace ,cloves, and sticks of cinnamon, with two nutmegs beaten small. And so serve it.

TO BOIL TEALS, MALLARDS, PIGEONS, CHINES OF PORK OR NEAT'S TONGUES, ALL AFTER ONE SORT

Let them be half roasted, stick a few cloves in their breasts, then two or three toasts of bread being burned black. Then put them into a little fair water: immediately take them out again, and strain them with a little wine and vinegar to the quantity of a pint. Put it into an earthen pot, and take eight or ten onions sliced small, being fried in a frying pan with a dish of butter. When they be fried, put them into your broth. Then take your meat from the spit and put it into the same broth, and so let them boil together for a time, seasoning with salt and pepper.

MUTTON BOILED FOR SUPPER

First set your mutton on the fire, skim it clean, then take out all the broth, leaving so much as will cover it. Then take and put thereto ten or twelve onions, peeled, cut them in quarters, with a handful of parsley, chopped fine, putting it to the mutton, and so let them boil. Season it with pepper, salt and saffron, with two or three spoonfuls of vinegar.

TO BOIL MUTTON WITH NAVENS*

First peel your navens, and wash them. Then cut five or six of them them into pieces to the bigness of an inch. And when your Mutton hath boiled a while take out all the liquor, saving so much as may cover well the mutton. Put your navens into the pot of mutton with a handful of parsley, chopped fine, and a branch of rosemary, seasoning it with salt and pepper and saffron.

* *A kind of turnip.*

TO BOIL A LAMB'S HEAD WITH PURTENANCES

First skim it well. Take of the broth, leaving so much as will cover it. Then put to it parsley and rosemary, a branch of hyssop and thyme, and a dish of butter, with barberries or gooseberries. Then let them boil, being seasoned with cloves, mace, salt, pepper, and saffron. And so serve it forth upon sops.

TO BOIL A CAPON IN WHITE BROTH

Take a well fleshed capon and a marrow bone, and a quart of fair water. Put them together in an earthen pot, and let them boil till the capon be enough. But you must take away the marrow from the bone. When it hath boiled, take the uppermost of the broth and put it into an earthen pot and the marrow with it. Put to it small raisins, prunes, whole mace, dates, and half a quartern of sugar, six spoonfuls of verjuice, and three or four yolks of eggs. Put these all chopped small, and three or four hard roasted eggs, being chopped with bread and suet, then a little water put too, and saffron. Colour it with three or four raw eggs, both yolks and whites, salt, pepper, cloves and mace being minced together, putting it into the mugget. And so boil it with a little mutton broth and wine, lettuce and spinach whole in the same broth. And so serve it forth.

TO BOIL MUTTON FOR SUPPER

Take carrot roots and cut them an inch long. Take a handful of parsley and thyme, half chopped, and put into a pot the mutton. So let them boil, being seasoned with salt and pepper, and so serve it forth.

TO BOIL A NEAT'S TONGUE FOR SUPPER

Take a little wine or fair water, putting unchopped lettuce, fair washed, into your neat's tongue, with a dish of butter or two. Season it with salt and pepper, cloves and mace. And so serve it.

TO BOIL MALLARDS, TEALS, AND CHINES OF PORK, WITH CABBAGE

First unloose your cabbage, and cut them in three or four quarters, unloosing every leaf, for doubt of worms to be in there. Then wash them and put them in a pot of fair water, and let them boil a quarter of an hour. Then take them up, and chop them somewhat great. Then put them into a fair pot with the broth of the mallard and whole pepper, and pepper beaten with cloves, mace, and salt. And so let them boil together etc.

21

after that but serve it forth upon sops. You may make balls after the same sort.

TO BOIL A BREAST OF VEAL OR
MUTTON, FARCED

Take a breast of veal or mutton and farce it in like manner as your cabbage is, so that you leave out the prunes and great raisins. Boil your veal or mutton in the aforesaid broths, putting no more broth than will cover your meat. And when your meat is half boiled, then put two handfuls of lettuce or spinach, cutting it four times asunder and no more. When your meat and herbs be boiled, then put a little verjuice in the broth. Season it with salt and pepper. Then serve your meat upon sops, casting your herbs upon it. And so serve it.

TO MAKE MUGGETS*

First parboil them, and take white and chop them both together, and put currants, dates, cinnamon and ginger, cloves and mace, and gross pepper, and sugar if you will, two or three yolks of eggs, and seethe them altogether with salt. Put the stuff into the cauls of mutton. And so put them in dishes, and take two or three eggs, white and all, and put them on the cauls. Make some pretty sauce for them.
* *Intestines of Calves or Sheep. This dish survives as faggots.*

TO BOIL A MUGGET OF SHEEP

First wash and scour it clean then parboil it a little. Then chop a piece of a kidney of mutton, small, and put it into a platter. Put the quantity of a farthing loaf, grated, with prunes and raisins, of each a handful, parsley and thyme, together, and when your capon is boiled, lay him in a fair platter; pour your broth upon him, and so serve him.

TO BOIL CHICKENS

Boil them as the lambs head and purtenance is boiled. And when you are to serve them, strain three or four yolks of eggs with verjuice, and put it into the pot and let it boil no more after the eggs be put in. Season it with salt, pepper,mace,and cloves, and so serve them. Thus may you boil a conie or muggets of veal as the chickens are boiled.

TO BOIL CHICKENS WITH SPINACH AND LETTUCE

Take a platter of spinach and lettuce and wash them clean, and when the pot is skimmed then put them in with a dish of butter, and a branch of rosemary with a little verjuice, being seasoned with salt and ginger, beaten.

TO MAKE PEARS TO BE BOILED IN MEAT

Take a piece of a leg of mutton or veal raw, being mixed with a little sheep's suet, and half a manchet grated fine, taking four raw egg yolks and al. Then take a little thyme, and parsley chopped small, a few gooseberries or barberries, or green grapes being whole. Put all these together, being seasoned with salt, saffron and cloves, beaten and wrought altogether. Then make rolls or balls like to a pear, and when you have so done, take the stalk of the sage, and put it into the ends of your pears or balls. Then take the fresh broth of beef, mutton, or veal, being put in to an earthen pot, putting the pears or balls in the same broth with salt, cloves, mace, and saffron. When you be ready to serve him, put two or three yolks of eggs into the broth. Let them boil no more.

TO BOIL CALVE'S FEET

Take a pint of white wine and a small quantity of water and small raisins and whole mace. Boil them together in a little verjuice, yolks of eggs mingled with them, and a piece of sweet butter. So serve them upon bread, sliced.

TO BOIL CHICKENS AND MUTTON AFTER THE DUTCH FASHION

First take chickens and mutton and boil them in water a good while; let a good deal of the water be boiled away. Then take out the mutton and chickens and the broth, [and] make white broth. Put in thereto cinnamon and ginger, sugar, a little pepper, a little verjuice, and a little flour to thicken it, and a little saffron. Take rosemary, thyme, marjoram, pennyroyal, hyssop, and half a dish of butter with a little salt. The liquor must be cold before the chickens be put in.

TO MAKE A BOILED MEAT AFTER THE FRENCH WAYS

Take pigeons and lard them, and then put them on a broach*. Let them be half roasted. Then take them off the broach and make a pudding of sweet herbs of every sort, a good handful, and chop ox white amongst the herbs, very small. Take the yolks of five or six eggs and grated bread, and season it with pepper, cinnamon and ginger, cloves and mace, sugar, and currants, and mingle altogether. Then put the stuff on the pigeons round about. Then put the pigeons into the cabbages, that be parboiled, and bind the cabbage fast to the pigeons. Then put them into the pot where you mean to boil them. Put in beef broth into them, and
*Spit.

cabbages chopped small, and so let them boil. Put in pepper, cloves and mace, and prick the pigeons full of cloves before you put the pudding on them. And put a piece of butter, cinnamon, and ginger, and put a little vinegar and white wine. And so serve them up and garnish them with fruit. And serve one in a dish, and but a little of the broth you must put into the dish when you serve them up.

TO BOIL THE LIGHTS* OF A CALF

First boil the lights in water. Then take parsley, thyme, onions, pennyroyal, and a little rosemary. When the lights be boiled chop all these together, lights and all, very small. Then boil them in a little pot, and put into them verjuice, butter, and some of their own broth. Then season it with pepper, cinnamon, and ginger. Let them boil a little and serve them with sops.
* *The lungs of an animal.*

TO BOIL NEAT'S FEET

Take your neat's feet out of the sauce* and wash them in fair water. Then put them into your mutton broth, and take five or six onions, chopped not small. Then take a quantity of thyme, parsley and hyssop, chopped fine. Boil all together, and when it is half boiled and more, then take a dish or two of butter, and put to it. Then season it with pepper, salt and saffron, with five or six spoonfuls of vinegar, and so serve it upon sops.
* *Brine.*

TO BOIL DIVERS KINDS OF FISH

Bret, conger, thornback, plaice, fresh salmon; all these you must boil with a little fair water and vinegar, a little salt, and bay leaves, and a little of the broth they are sodden in with a little salt. As you see cause, shift your sauce, as you do beef in brine, and also fresh sturgeon. Seethe it as aforesaid and sauce it as you did the other. And so you may keep it half a year with changing of the sauce. Salt sturgeon; seethe it in water and salt, and a little vinegar. Let it be cold and serve it forth with vinegar, and a little fennel upon it, but first ere you seethe it, it must be watered.

TO BOIL A BREAM

Take white wine and put it into a pot and let it seethe. Then take your bream and cut him in the midst and put him in. Take an onion and chop it small. Then take nutmegs beaten, cinnamon and ginger, whole mace, and a pound of butter and let it boil together. So season it with salt, serve it upon sops, and garnish with fruit.

TO BOIL MUSSELS

Take water and yeast, a good dish of butter, and onions, chopt, and a little pepper. When it hath boiled a little while, see that your mussels be clean washed, then put them into the broth, shells and all. And when they be boiled well serve them broth and all.

TO BOIL STOCKFISH*

Take stockfish when it is well watered and pick out all the best [parts] clean from the fish. Then put it into a pipkin
* *Often Haddock or Cod, dried. Sometimes kept alive in water.*

and put in no more water than shall cover it, and set it on the fire. As soon as it beginneth to boil on the one side then turn the other side to the fire, and soon as it beginneth to boil on the side take it off and put it into a collander. Let the water run out from it, but put in salt in the boiling of it. Then take a little fair water and sweet butter, and let it boil in a dish until it be something thick. Then pour it on the stockfish and serve it.

TO SEETHE A CARP

First take a carp and boil it in water and salt. Then take of the broth and put it in a little pot. Then put thereto as much wine as there is broth, with rosemary, parsley, thyme, and marjoram bound together. Put them into the pot. Put thereto a good many of sliced onions, small raisins, whole maces, a dish of butter, and a little sugar, so that it be not too sharp nor too sweet. Let all these seethe together. If the wine be not sharp enough then put thereto a little vinegar. And so serve it upon sops with broth.

TO SEETHE A PIKE

First seethe the pike in water and salt, with rosemary, parsley, and thyme. Then take the best of the broth and put [it] into a litle pot. Put thereto the ruffilt* of the pike, small raisins, whole mace, whole pepper, twelve or thirteen dates, a good piece of butter, a goblet of white wine, and a little yeast. When they have boiled a good while put in a little vinegar, sugar, and ginger. So serve the pike with the ruffilt and broth upon sops.
* *Possibly a misspelling of refect.*

TO SEETHE MUSSELS

Take butter and vinegar, a good deal, parsley, chopped small, and pepper. Then set it on the fire and let it boil a while. Then see the Mussels be clean washed, and put them in the broth shells and all. When they be boiled a while, serve them shells and all.

TO BOIL A CARP

Take out the gall, cast it away, and so scald not your carp nor yet wash him. When you do kill him let his blood fall into a platter, and split your carp into the same blood and cast thereon a ladleful of vinegar. Then toast three or four toasts of brown bread, and burn it black, and dip them into a little fair water. Immediately strain them into the liquor where your carp shall be sodden, with three or four onions chopped somewhat big, with parsley chopped small. Then set your broth upon the fire, and when it begins to boil, put to your carp two or three dishes of butter and a branch of rosemary, slipped, and slips of thyme. If it be too thick put to it a little wine; and so let it boil fair and softly, seasoning it with whole mace, cloves and salt, and pepper, cloves and mace, beaten. And so serve him.

TO BOIL A PIKE ANOTHER WAY

Take your pike and pull out all his guts, and do not split your pike, but cut off his head, whole, and cut his body in three or four pieces. And so let him be boiled in wine, water and salt, to the quantity of a pottel. Then take a pint of wine and a ladleful or two of the pike's broth, and put these together into an earthen pot, with two dishes of butter, and three or four oranges, sliced, small raisins, and sugar, thyme, and rosemary, slipped. And then put in the effect* of the

* *Possibly a misspelling of refect, a portion.*

pike in the same broth, and so let them boil together. And when you be ready to serve, lay your pike upon sops, and put your broth upon it, seasoning it with whole cinnamon, mace, and a nutmeg, beaten. And so serve it forth.

TO BOIL ROACH, PERCH, AND DACE, AND OTHER SMALL FISH

Take fair water and put to it parsley, thyme, and rosemary, slipped; let it boil a good while together. Then take a dish or two of butter, putting [it] to the same broth and your fish, and so let it boil together; seasoning it with cloves, mace, pepper, and salt. And so serve them upon sops.

TO BOIL PIKE ANOTHER WAY

Take and split your pike through the back and take out the refect.* So done, put your pike into a pan of water with rosemary. Let it seethe till it be boiled. Then take your reject with a little wine and verjuice, with two dishes of butter, put these in a platter, setting it on a chafing dish of coals. There let it boil, seasoning it with whole mace. This done, take up your pike, laying him upon sops on a platter. Then take your refect and his broth and cast upon it, and so serve it forth with salt.

* *Portion, possibly the roe and liver.*

TO BOIL A TENCH

Seethe your tench with a little water and a good deal of vinegar. When it is sodden lay it in a fair dish, take out all the bones, and put a little saffron in your broth with a little salt. Put the same broth upon your tench, and cast a little fine pepper upon it while it is hot. And so let your tench stand till it be on a jelly. When you do serve it take an onion and parsley, chopped fine, and cast it upon your tench and so serve it.

FOR TURBOT AND CONGER

Seethe them in fair water and salt and let them boil till they be enough. Then take them from the fire and let them cool. Then use them in the seasoning as the salmon hereafter following.

FOR FRESH SALMON

Take your salmon and boil him in fair water, rosemary and thyme; and in the seething put a quart of strong ale to it. And so let it boil till it be enough. Then take it from the fire, and let it cool. Then take your salmon out of the pan and put it into an earthen pan or wooden bowl, and there put so much broth as will cover him. Put into the same broth a good deal of vinegar, so that it be tart with it.

TO BOIL COCKLES

Take water, vinegar, pepper, and beer, and put the cockles in it. Then let them seethe a good while and serve them broth and all. You may seethe them in nothing but in water and salt if you will.

TO BOIL A CARP IN GREEN BROTH WITH
A PUDDING IN HIS BELLY

Take the spawn of a carp, and boil and crumble it as fine as you can. Then take grated bread, small raisins, dates minced, cinnamon, sugar, cloves, mace, pepper and a little salt, mingled altogether. Take a good handful of sage and boil it tender, and strain it with three or four yolks of eggs, and one white. Put [it] to the spawn with a little cream and rose water. Then take the carp and put the pudding in the belly and seethe him in water and salt. When he is almost boiled take some of the spawn and of the best of the broth, and put it into a little pot with a little white wine, a good piece of butter, three or four onions, whole mace, whole pepper, small raisins,and three or four dates. When it is a good deal sodden, put in a good deal of seeded spinach, and strain it with three or four yolks of eggs, and the onions that you put into your broth with a little verjuice, and put to your broth. If it be too sharp put in a little sugar. And so lay your carp upon sops and pour the broth upon it.

TO DRESS A CARP

Take your carp and scale it and split it, and cut off his head, and take out all the bones from him clean. Then take the fish and mince it fine, being raw, with the yolks of four or five hard eggs minced with it. So done, put it into an earthen pot with two dishes of butter and a pint of white wine, a handful of prunes, [and] two yolks of hard eggs cut in four quarters. Season it with one nutmeg, not small beaten, salt, cinnamon, and ginger. And in the boiling of it you must stir it that it burn not to the pot bottom. When it is enough, then take your minced meat and lay it in the dish, making the proportion of the body, setting his head at the upper end and his tail at the lower end: which head and tail must be sodden by themselves in a vessel with water and salt.

You may use a pike thus in all points, so that you do not take the prunes, but for them take dates and small raisins. When you have seasoned it as your carp is, and when you do serve it, put the refect into the pike's mouth, gaping, and so serve it forth.

TO BOIL ONIONS

Take a good many onions and cut them in four quarters. Set them on the fire in as much water as you think will boil them tender. When they be clean skimmed, put in a good many small raisins, half a spoonful of gross pepper, a good piece of sugar, and a little salt. When the onions be thorough boiled, beat the yolk of an egg with verjuice, and put into your pot. So serve it upon sops. If you will, poach eggs and lay upon them.

TO BOIL CITRONS

When your citrons be boiled, pared and sliced, seethe them with water and wine. Put to them butter, small raisins, barberries, sugar, cinnamon and ginger. Let them seethe till your citrons be tender.

TO MAKE A WHITE BROTH WITH ALMONDS

First look that your meat be clean washed, and then set it on the fire and when it boileth skim it clean. Put some salt into the pot. Then take rosemary and thyme, hyssop and marjoram, and bind them together and put them into the pot. Take a dish of sweet butter and put it into the pot amongst your meat. And take some whole mace and bind them in a cloth, and put them into the pot with a quantity of verjuice. After that take a quantity of almonds as shall serve the turn, blanch them, and beat them in a mortar, and then strain them with the broth your meat is in. When these almonds are strained put them in a pot by themselves with some sugar, a little ginger, and also a little rose water. Then stir it while [it] boil. After that take some sliced oranges, without the kernels, and boil them with the broth of the pot upon a chafing dish of coal with a little sugar. Then have some sippets ready in a platter and serve the meat upon them. Put not your almonds in till it be ready to be served.

FOR WHITE PEASE POTTAGE

Take a quart of white pease or more, and seethe them in fair water, close, until they do cast all their husks, the white cast away as long as any will come up to the top. And when they be gone; then put into the pease two dishes of butter, and a little verjuice, with pepper and salt, and a little fine powder of march.* And so let it stand till you will occupy it, and then serve it upon sops. You may seethe the porpoise and seal in your pease, serving it forth two pieces in a dish.
* *Pulverised spices.*

TO MAKE STEWED STEAKS

Take a piece of mutton and cut it in pieces and wash it very clean. Put it into a fair pot with ale, or half wine. Then make it boil and skim it clean. Put into your pot a faggot of rosemary and thyme. Then take some parsley picked fine, and some onions cut round, and let them all boil together. Then take prunes and raisins, dates and currants, and let it boil altogether. Season it with cinnamon and ginger, nutmegs, two or three cloves, and salt. And so serve it on sops and garnish it with fruit.

TO STEW CALVE'S FEET

Take calve's feet, fair blanched, and cut them in the half. When they be more than half boiled, put to them great raisins, mutton broth, a little saffron and sweet butter, pepper, sugar and some sweet herbs, finely minced. Boil calve's feet, sheep's feet, or lambs' feet, with mutton broth, sweet herbs and onions chopped fine, butter and pepper. When they boil take the yolk of an egg and strain it with verjuice. So serve it.

TO STEW A MALLARD

Take your mallard and seethe him in fair water, with a good marrow bone, and cabbagewort, or cabbage lettuce, or both, or some parsnip roots and carrot roots. When all these be well sodden, put in prunes enough and three dates, and season him with salt, cloves and mace, and a little sugar and pepper. Then serve it forth with sippets and put the marrow upon them, and the whole mace lay on the sippets. The dates quartered and the prunes, and the roots cut in round slices, lay upon the sippets also, and the cabbage leaves lay upon the Mallard.

TO STEW A COCK

You must cut him in five pieces and wash him clean. Take prunes, currants and dates cut very small, and raisins of the sun,* and sugar beaten very small, cinnamon, ginger and nutmegs, likewise beaten, and a little maydens,** cut very small. You must put him in a pipkin and put in almost a pint of muscadine, and then your spice and sugar upon your cock. Put in your fruit between every quarter, and a piece of gold*** between every piece of your cock. Then you must make a lid of wood to fit for your pipkin, and close it as close as you can with paste that no air come out, nor water can come in. Then you must fill two brass pots full of water and set on the fire. Make fast the pipkin in one of the brass pots, so that the pipkins feet touch not the brass pot's bottom, nor the pot sides. So let them boil four and twenty hours. Fill up the pot still as it boils away with the other pot that stands by. When it is boiled take out your gold, and let him drink it, fasting; and it shall help him. This is approved.

* *Genuine dried raisins, as apart from dried currants.*
** *Apples.*
*** *Pieces of gold leaf.*

TO STEW A CAPON FOR DINNER

Take a knuckle of veal and boil it with your capon, putting to it prunes, raisins great and small, whole mace, and let it boil together, seasoning it with salt, and so serve it forth.

TO STEW OYSTERS

Take your oysters and put them either in a little skillet over the fire,or else in a platter over a chafing dish of coals. And so let them boil with their liquor, sweet butter, verjuice, vinegar, and pepper, and of the tops of thyme, a little; till they be enough. Then serve them upon sops.

TO STEW VEAL

Take a knuckle of veal and bruise it. Then set it on the fire in a little fresh water and let it seethe a good while. Then take [a] good plenty of onions, and chop them into your broth. When it hath well sodden, put in verjuice, butter, salt and saffron. When it is enough, put to it a little sugar and then it will be good.

TO STEW STEAKS

Take a neck of mutton and cut it in pieces. Then fry them with butter until they be more than half enough. Fry them with a good many onions, sliced. Put them in a little pot, and put thereto a little parsley, chopped, as much broth of mutton or beef as may cover them with a little pepper, salt, and verjuice. Then let it seethe together very softly the space of an hour. Serve them upon sops.

TO STEW STEAKS

Take the great ribs of a neck of mutton and chop them asunder and wash them well. Then put them in a platter, one by another, and set them on a chafing dish of coals. Cover them and turn them now and then. So let them stew till they be half enough. Then take parsley and thyme, marjoram and onions, and chop them very small and cast upon the steaks. Put thereto one spoonful of verjuice, two or three spoonfuls of wine, [and] a little butter and marrow. Let them boil till the mutton be tender. Cast thereon a little pepper. If your broth be too sharp put in a little sugar.

ROASTING

FRYING

FRITTERS

PUDDINGS

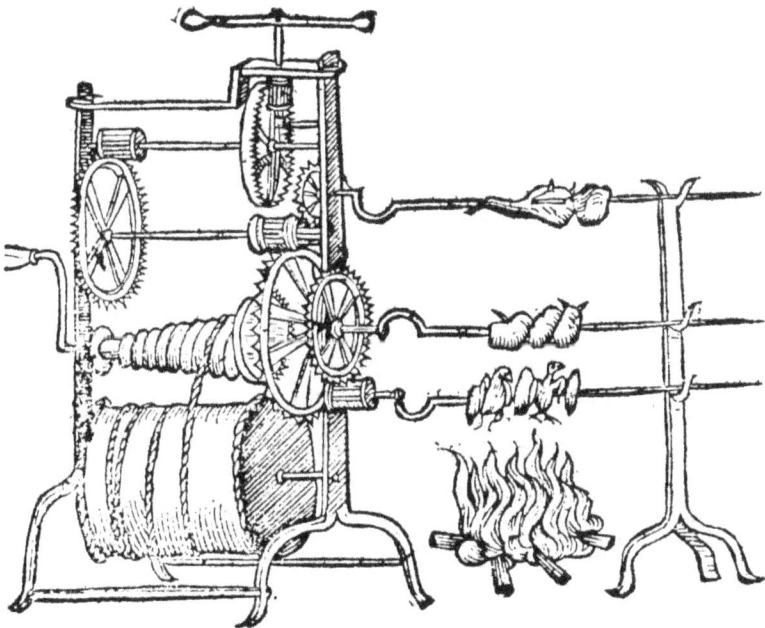

TO ROAST A CARP OR TENCH WITH A PUDDING
IN HIS BELLY

Take the rones* of a pyke and chop them very small. Then put in grated bread, two or three eggs, currants, dates, sugar, cinnamon ginger, mace, pepper and salt, and put it in his belly. Put him on a broche**, and make sweet sauce with barberries, or lemons, minced, and put into the sweet sauce. Then put it on the carp when you serve it up.

* *Roe.*
** *Spit.*

TO DRESS A HARE

Wash her in fair water, parboil her, then lay her in cold water. Then lard her and roast her. For sauce take red wine, salt, vinegar, ginger, pepper,cloves and mace,and put these together. Then mince onions and apples and fry them in a pan. Then put your sauce to them with a little sugar. And let them boil together and so serve it.

TO ROAST DEER'S TONGUES

Take deer's tongues and lard them and serve them with sweet sauce.

TO ROAST A LAMB'S HEAD

Take a head and purtenances, being clean washed. Cut the purtenances in pieces, so that it may be broached, and roast them, basting it with butter. When it is enough take the yolks of two raw eggs, with a little parsley, chopped fine, beating them together, and baste your lambs head with it, even so long till your eggs be hardened on. Then take it up, and serve it with the sauce of pepper, vinegar, and butter, boiled a little upon a chafing dish of coals.

TO MAKE ALOES TO ROAST OR BOIL

Take a leg of mutton and slice it thin. Then take out the kidneys of the mutton, having it minced small, with hyssop,thyme, parsley, and the yolks of hard eggs. Then bind it with crumbs of white bread and raw eggs, and put to it prunes, and great raisins, and for want of them, barberries, gooseberries, or grapes: seasoning it with cloves, mace, pepper, cinnamon, ginger and salt. You may make a mugget of a sheep as these aloes be, saving you must put no mutton in to it.

TO ROAST A PIG

Take your pig and draw it and wash it clean. Take the liver, parboil it and strain it with a little cream and yolks of eggs. Put thereto grated bread, marrow, small raisins, nutmegs in powder, mace, sugar and salt, and stir all these together, and put into the pig's belly, and sew the pig. Then spit it with the hair on. When it is half enough, pull off the skin; take heed you take not of the fat; then baste it. When it is enough,then crumb it with white bread, sugar, cinnamon, and ginger, and let it be somewhat brown.

TO ROAST AN HARE

Take the hare and flay her. Then take parsley, thyme, savory, cream, a good piece of butter, pepper, small raisins, and barberries. Work all these together in the hare's belly. When she is almost enough, baste her with butter and one yolk of an egg. Make venison sauce to her.

TO ROAST A HARE

You must not cut off her head, feet, nor ears, but make a pudding in her belly. Put paper about her ears that they burn not. When the hare is roasted, you must take cinnamon, ginger, and grated bread, and you must make very sweet sauce. And you must put in barberries and let them boil together.

TO FRY CHICKEN

Take your chickens and let them boil in very good sweet broth a pretty while. Take the chickens out and quarter them out in pieces. Then put them into a frying pan with sweet butter, and let them stew in the pan. But you must not let them be brown with frying. Then put out the butter out of the pan, and then take a little sweet broth, and as much verjuice, and the yolks of two eggs and beat them together. Put in a little nutmeg, cinnamon, ginger, and pepper into the sauce. Then put them all into the pan to the chickens, and stir them together in the pan. Put them into a dish and serve them up.

TO FRY BACON

Take bacon and slice it very thin and cut away the lean and bruise it with the back of your knife. Fry it in sweet butter and serve it.

TO MAKE FRITTERS OF SPINACH

Take a good deal of spinach and wash it clean. Then boil it in fair water. When it is boiled take it forth and let the water run from it. Then chop it with the back of a knife, and put in some eggs and grated bread. Season it with sugar, cinnamon, ginger and pepper, dates minced fine, and currants. Roll them like a ball and dip them in batter made of ale and flour.

A FRITTER TO BE MADE IN A MOULD

Take ox white* and mince it fine, then take dates and mince them fine. Then take currants, eggs, white grated bread, and season it with sugar, cinnamon, ginger, cloves, mace and saffron, and stir it well together. Then drive* a thick cake of paste and lay [it] in the mould. Fill it with the stuff and lay another cake of paste upon it. Then jog it about, and so fry it.
* *Flank of Beef.*
** *Roll out.*

TO MAKE FRITTER STUFF

Take fine flour, and three or four eggs, put into the flour, and a piece of butter, and let them boil altogether in a dish or a chafer. Put in sugar, cinnamon and ginger, and rose water. And in the boiling put in a little grated bread to make it big. Then put it into a dish and beat it well together. And so put it into your mould and fry it with clarified butter. But your butter may not be too hot or too cold.

TO MAKE A VAUNT*

Take marrow of beef, as much as you can hold in both hands, cut it as big as great dice.   Then take dates and cut them as big as small dice. Then take forty prunes and cut the fruit from the stones. Then take half a handful of small raisins, wash them clean and prick them, and put your marrow in a fair platter, and your dates, prunes, and small raisins. Then take twenty yolks of eggs and put in your stuff before rehearsed. Then take a quartern of sugar or more, and beat it small, and put in your marrow. Then take two spoonfuls of cinnamon and a spoonful of ginger, and put them to your stuff and mingle them altogether. Then take eight yolks of eggs and four spoonfuls of rose water, strain them, and put a little sugar in it. Then take a fair frying pan and put in a little piece of butter, as much as a walnut, and set it upon a good fire. And when it looketh almost black, put it out of your pan, and as fast as you can put half of your eggs in the midst of your pan and fry it yellow. When it is fried put it into a fair dish and put your stuff therein. Spread it all [over] the bottom of your dish. Then make another vaunt even as you made the other. Set it upon a fair board, cut it in pretty pieces of the length of your will finger, as long as your vaunt is, and lay it upon your stuff after the fashion of a little window. Then cut off the ends of them as much as lieth without the inward compass of the dish. Then set the dish within the oven, or in a baking pan, and let it bake with leisure. When it is baked enough, the marrow will come fair out of the vaunt to the brim of the dish. Then draw it out and cast a little sugar on it, and so serve it in.

* *A type of fritter.*

TO MAKE A PUDDING IN A BREAST OF VEAL

Take parsley and thyme, wash them, prick them and chop them small. Then take eight yolks of eggs, grated bread, and half a pint of cream being very sweet. Then season it with pepper, cloves and mace, saffron and sugar, small raisins and salt. Put it in and roast it and serve it.

TO MAKE A PUDDING OF A
CALVES CHALDRON*

First take the chaldron and let it be washed and scalded and parboiled. Let it be chopped and stamped fine in a mortar. While it is hot strain it through a collander; and half a dozen of eggs, both whites and yolks, with all manner of herbs, to them a handful or two. Let the herbs be shred small, and put them to the chaldron, and a good handful of grated bread. Then take a handful of flour and put it to it all. Then take an orange peel out of the syrup and mingle with it. Then season it with cinnamon and ginger, and a few cloves and mace, a little rose water, and marrow or suet. Butter a good quantity thereof and close it up so it be not dry baked. Then take the thinnest of sheep's caul and wrap the meat in [it]. Then raise the coffin of fine paste and put it in.
* Or *chaudron, entrails.*

TO MAKE BLACK PUDDING

Take great oatmeal and lay it in milk to steep. Then take sheep's blood and put to it, and take ox white and mince into it. Then take a few sweet herbs and two or three leek blades and chop tjem very small. Then put into it the yolks of some eggs, and season it with cinnamon, ginger, cloves, mace, pepper and salt. And so fill them.

TO MAKE A HAGGIS PUDDING

Take a piece of calves chaldron and parboil it. Shred it so small as you can. Then take as much beef suet as your meat, shred likewise, and a good deal more of grated bread. Put this together, and [add] to them seven or eight yolks of eggs, two or three whites, a little cream, three or four spoonfuls of rose water, a little pepper, mace and nutmegs, and a good deal of sugar. Fill them and let them be sodden with a very soft fire. Shred also with a little winter savory, parsley and thyme, and a little pennyroyal, with your meat.

TO MAKE A HOG'S PUDDING

Take the liver of a hog and parboil it. Then stamp [it] in water and strain it with thick cream. Put thereto eight or nine yolks of eggs, three or four whites, hog's suet, small raisins, cloves and mace, pepper, salt and a little sugar, and a good deal of grated bread to make it thick. And let them seethe.

TO MAKE A PUDDING

Take parsley and thyme and chop it small. Then take the kidney of veal, and parboil it, and when it is parboiled, take all the fat off it, and lay it that it may cool. When it is cold shred it like as you do suet for puddings. Then take marrow and mince it by itself. Then take grated bread and small raisins the quantity of your stuff, and dates minced small. Then take the eggs and roast them hard and take the yolks of them and chop them small, and them take your stuff aforerehearsed, and mingle altogether. Then take pepper, cloves and mace, saffron, and salt, and put it together with the said stuff, as much as you think by casting shall suffice. Then take six eggs and break them into a vessel, whites and all. Put your dry stuff into the same eggs, and temper them all well together. So fill your haggis or gut, and seethe it well and it will be good.

TO MAKE A PUDDING IN A POT

Take a piece of a leg of mutton or veal, and parboil it well. Then shred it very fine with as much suet as there is mutton. Season it with a little pepper and salt, cloves and mace, with a good deal of cinnamon and ginger. Then put it in a little pot, and put thereto a good quantity of currants and prunes, and two or three dates cut long ways. Let it seethe softly with a little verjuice, upon sops. So serve it with sugar.

TO SMOTHER A CONEY

Take the livers and boil them and chop them. [Add] sweet herbs, apples, and the yolks of hard eggs, and chop them altogether with currants, sugar, cinnamon, ginger, and parsley, and fill the coney full thereof. Then put her into the sweet broth and put in sweet butter. Chop the yolks of hard eggs, cinnamon, and sugar, and cast it on the coney when you serve it up. Season it with salt, serve it on sops, and garnish with fruit.

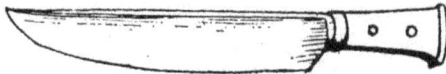

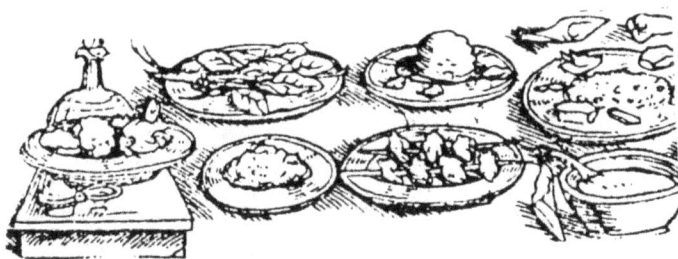

MISCELLANEOUS

SAVOURY

RECIPES

TO MAKE A SAUSAGE

Take Martinmass* beef, or if you can not get it, take fresh beef, or the lean of bacon if you will. You must mince very small that kind of flesh that you take. And cut lard and put it into the minced meat, and whole pepper, and the yolks of seven eggs, and mingle them altogether. And cut the meat into a gut very salt, and hang him in the chimney where he may dry. There let him hang a month or two before you take him down.
* *Salt beef.*

TO MAKE A MORTISE*

Take almonds and blanch them and beat them in a mortar. Boil a chicken and take the flesh of him and beat it and strain them together with milk and water. And so put them into a pot and put in sugar and stir them still. When it hath boiled a good while, take it off and set it acooling in a pail of water. Strain it again with rose water into a dish.
* *A dish of pounded meat.*

TO MAKE MORTISE OF A CAPON, HEN, OR PULLET

Take a well fleshed capon, hen, or pullet; scald and dress him. Then put him into a pot of fair water, and there let it seethe till it be tender. Then take it and pull all the flesh from his bones, and beat it in a stone mortar. And when you think it half beaten, put some of the same liquor into it, and then beat it till it be fine. Then take it out and strain it with a little rosewater out of a strainer into a dish. Then take it and set it on a chafing dish of coals, with a little sugar put to it, and so stir it with your knife. Lay it in a fair dish in three long rows. Then take blanch powder made of cinnamon and sugar, and cast upon it, and so serve it forth.

TO MAKE ALOES*

Take a leg of veal or mutton, and slice it in thin slices. Lay them in a platter and cast on salt. Put thereon the yolks of ten eggs and a great sort of small raisins and dates, finely minced. Then take vinegar and a little saffron, cloves and mace, and a little pepper, and mingle it together and pour it all about it. Then also work it together, and when it is thoroughly seasoned put it on a spit and set platters underneath it. Baste it with butter and make a sauce with vinegar, ginger, and sugar. Lay the aloes upon it. So serve it in.

* *Any dish made with sliced meats.*

TO MAKE ALOES

Take a leg of mutton or veal, and cut it in thin slices. Take parsley, thyme, marjoram, savory, and chop them small with two or three yolks of hard eggs. Put thereto a good many currants. Then put these herbs in the slices, with a piece of butter in each of them. Wrap them together and lay them close in your paste. Season them with cloves, mace, cinnamon, sugar and a little whole pepper, currants and barberries cast upon them. And put a dish of butter to them. When they be almost baked, put in a little verjuice.

TO MAKE ALOES OF FRESH SALMON
TO BOIL OR TO BAKE

Take your salmon and cut him small in pieces of three fingers breadth. And when you have cut so many slices as you will have, let them be of the length of a woman's hand.

Then take more of the salmon, as much as you think good, and mince it raw with six yolks of hard eggs, very fine: then two or dishes of butter, with small raisins, and so work them together with cloves, mace, pepper and salt. Then lay your minced meat in your sliced aloes, every one being rolled and pricked with a feather, full closed. Then put your aloes into an earthen pot. and put to it a pint of water, and another pint of claret wine, and so let them boil till they be enough. Afterward take the yolks of three raw eggs with a little verjuice, being strained together, and so put into the pot. Then let your aloes seethe no more afterward, but serve them upon sops of bread.

TO MAKE GOOSE GIBLETS AND PIG'S PETTITOES

Let them be sodden thoroughly, then cut them in pieces and fry them in butter. When they be half fried, then put to a little vinegar with ginger, cinnamon and pepper, and so serve it forth. Thus may you use calves feet boiled in all points as this.

FOR FRICASEES OF A LAMB'S HEAD AND PURTENANCE

Take a lamb's head and clean it, and cut his purtenances in pieces, and parboil it till it be almost enough. Then take the yolks of two raw eggs and baste your lamb's head and purtenance with it, and fry it in butter for sauce. Put to the butter, pepper,vinegar,and salt; frying them together a little on the fire, and so serve it.

FOR FRICASEES OF NEAT'S FEET FOR SUPPER

Take your neat's feet and clean them, and baste them with butter and crumbs of bread, and lay them upon a gridiron, till they be thoroughly broiled. Then take vinegar, pepper, and salt, and butter, and put them altogether in a dish. Set on a chafing dish of coals, boiling, and so let them boil there till you must serve it. You must put to sauce, barberries, grapes, etc.

A FRICASEE OF TRIPES

Let them be fair sodden, and sauce them. Take the leanest and cut in pieces, an inch broad. Fry them with butter or flattes;* and your sauce to be vinegar, pepper, and mustard, being put a little while in the frying pan with butter or flattes.
* *Lard.*

TO MAKE A RED DEER

Take a leg of beef and cut out all the sinews clean. Then take a rolling pin and all to beat it; then parboil it. And when you have so done, lard it very thick. Then lay it in wine or vinegar for two or three hours, or a whole night. Then take it out and season it with pepper, salt, cloves, and mace. Then put it into your paste, and so bake it.

TO FARCE ALL THINGS

Take a good handful of thyme, hyssop, and three or four yolks of eggs, hard roasted, and chop them with herbs, small. Then take white bread, grated, and raw eggs with sweet butter, a few small raisins or barberries; seasoning it with pepper, cloves, mace, cinnamon and ginger; working it altogether as paste. Then may you stuff with it what you will.

TO MAKE TOASTS

Take the kidney of veal and chop it small, then set it on a chafing dish of coals. Take two yolks of eggs, currants, cinnamon, ginger, cloves, mace, and sugar. Let them boil together a good while. Put a little butter with the kidney.

A MADE DISH OF THE PROPORTION OF
AN EGG FOR FLESH DAYS

Make in all your things your farcing stuff as you do for your cabbage, even so much as will fill a bladder. First take a bladder and dry it and wash it clean, that is of a calf or of a steer. Cut a little hole in the top and then put in all your farcing stuff. When you have filled it then close the bladder top, binding it with a thread. Put it into fresh beef broth, or mutton broth, and there let it seethe till it be enough. Then take it out, and let it stand till it be somewhat stiff. Then cut away the bladder from it. Take another dry bladder, and wash it clean, let it be bigger somewhat than the other was before; cut it broad at the top whereby your farcing stuff may in the hole go. When it is in, then put so many whites of eggs, being raw, as may run round about him, both above and beneath, within the bladder, clean covered with it. Then bind up your bladder mouth and put into your broth again the bladder. And there let it seethe till the white be hardened about the farcing, then take it out and cut away the bladder. Then set it in a fair dish, laying the parsley upon it, and so serve it forth.

Thus may you make small eggs to the number of six or eight in a dish in like manner, having a bladder for the same purpose.

TO FORCE A PIG

Take white wine and a little sweet broth, and half a score nutmegs cut in quarters. Then take rosemary, bays, thyme and sweet marjoram, and let them boil altogether. Skim them very clean and when they be boiled put them into an earthen pan, and the syrup also. And when you serve them, a quarter in a dish and the bays and nutmegs on the top.

TO MAKE BLAMEMANGLE*

Take all the brain of a capon and stamp it in a mortar, fine, and blanched almonds, and sometimes put to them rose water. Season it with powder of cinnamon, ginger, and sugar. And so serve it.
Literally, white food.

TO MAKE A FLORENTINE

Take the kidneys of a loin of veal that is roasted, and when it is cold, shred it fine, and grate, as it were, half a manchette,* very fine. Take eight yolks of eggs, and a handful of currants, and eight dates, finely shred, a little cinnamon, a little ginger,a little sugar, and a little salt, and mingle them with the kidneys. Then take a handful of fine flour and two yolks of eggs and as much butter as two eggs, and put into your flour. Then take a little seething liquor and make your paste and drive it abroad, very thin. Then stroke your dish with a little butter and lay your paste in a dish and fill it with your meat. Then draw another sheet of paste, thin, and cover it withal. Cut it handsomely upon the top and by the sides, and then put it into the oven.   And
* *Manchet rolls of best white bread are equal to 6oz. Two manchets make one loaf. The rolls are thick in the middle and sharp at the ends.*

when it is half baked draw it out, and take two or three feathers, and a little rose water, and wet all the cover with it. And have a handful of sugar finely beaten and strewn upon it. See that the rose water wet[s] every place, and so set it in the oven again, and that will make a fair ice upon it. If your oven be not hot enough to rear up your ice, then put a little fire in the oven's mouth.

TO KEEP LARD IN SEASON

Cut your lard in fair pieces and salt it well with white salt, every piece with your hand, and lay it in a close vessel. Then take fair running water, and much white salt in it, to make it brine. Then boil it until it bear an egg. Then put it into your lard and keep it close.

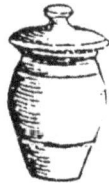

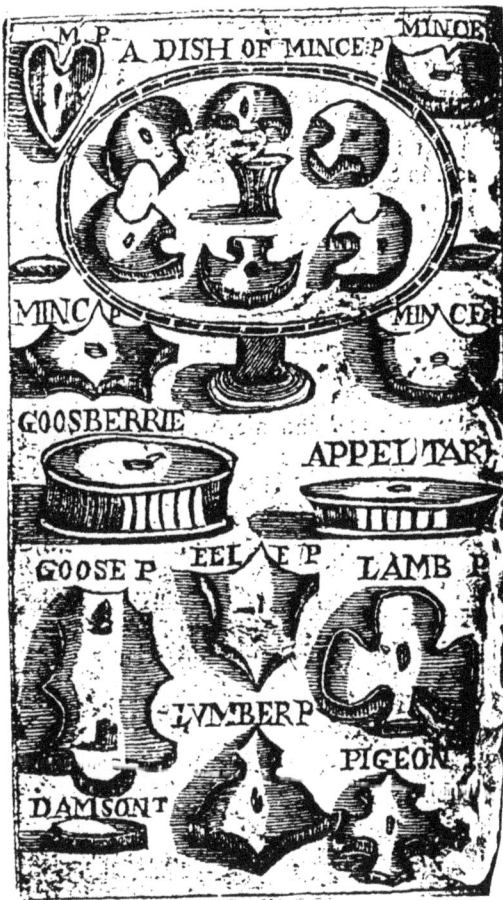

BAKING

TO MAKE A SYRUP FOR BAKE MEATS

Take ginger, cloves and mace, nutmegs [and] beat all these together very fine. Boil them in good red vinegar until it be somewhat thick. This being done, draw your pie when it is hard baked, and a small hole being made in the cover thereof at the first, with a funnel of paste, you must pour the syrup into the pie. That done, cover the hole with paste and shape the pie well and set it in the oven again till it be thoroughly baked. When you have drawn it, turn the bottom upward until it be served.

TO MAKE BAKE MEATS

Take a leg of Lamb, and cut out all the flesh and save the skin whole. Mince it fine and white* with it. Then put in grated bread and some eggs, white and all, and some dates and currants. Season it with some pepper, cinnamon, ginger, nutmeg and caraways, and a little cream, and temper it altogether. Then put it into the leg of lamb again and let it bake a little before you put it in your pie. When you have put it in your pie then put in a little of the pudding about it. When it is almost baked, then put in verjuice, sugar and sweet butter. And so serve it.
* *Flank.*

ANOTHER BAKE MEAT

Take a leg of veal and cut in slices and beat it with the back of a knife. Then take thyme, marjoram and pennyroyal, savory, and parsley, and one onion, and chop them all together very small. Then break in some eggs, whites and all, and put in your herbs and season it with pepper, nutmegs and salt, and a little sugar. Then stir them all together and lap them up like aloes. Cast a few currants and dates and butter amongst them.

ANOTHER BAKE MEAT

Take two pounds of white and a little veal and mince it together. Then take a little pennyroyal, savory and marjoram, and unset leeks and chop them fine. Put in some eggs and some cream. Then stir it all well together, and season it with pepper, nutmegs, and salt. Then put it into the pie and cut the lid and let it bake till it be dry. Then serve it.

TO MAKE FILLETS OF BEEF OR CLOD*
INSTEAD OF RED DEER

First take your beef and lard it very thick, and season it with pepper and salt, cinnamon and ginger, cloves and mace good store**, with a great deal more quantity of pepper and salt than you would a venison. Put it in covered paste. When it is baked take vinegar and sugar, cinnamon and ginger, and put [them] in, and shape the pasty and stop it close. Let it stand almost a fortnight before you cut it up.
* *The coarse part of an ox neck nearest the shoulder.*
** *Strongly.*

TO BAKE CONIES

Have fine paste ready. Wash your conies and parboil them. Then cast them into the cold water. Season them with salt and ginger. Lay them into the paste and upon them lay leached* lard, close them and bake them.
* *Sliced.*

TO BAKE A BREAST OF VEAL

Take and break the bones thereof in the middle and parboil him and take out the bones. Season him with pepper and salt and lay him in the coffin with a little sweet butter,

and close him up. Then make a caudle* of the yolk of an egg and strain it, and boil it in a chafing dish of coals. Season it with sugar, and put it in the pie and set it into the oven again.**
* *Gruel.*
** *This pie must have been put into the oven after it was first closed.*

TO BAKE A GAMMON OF BACON

Take a gammon of bacon, water it five days, and parboil him half enough and lay him in paste. Then take the sworde* of him and stuff him with cloves and season him with pepper and saffron. Close up in a standing pie. Bake him, and so serve him.
* *Rind.*

TO BAKE A TURKEY AND TAKE OUT HIS BONES

Take a fat turkey, and after you have scalded him and washed him clean, lay him upon a fair cloth and slit him throughout the back. When you have taken out his garbage then you must take out his bones so bare as you can. When you have so done wash him clean. Then truss him and prick his back together. And so have a fair kettle of seething water and parboil him a little. Then take him up that the water may run clean out of him. When he is cold, season him with pepper and salt. Then prick him with a few cloves in the breast, and also draw him with lard if you like of it. When you have made of your coffin and laid your turkey in it, so then you must put some butter in it, and close him up. In this sort you may bake a goose, a pheasant or capon.

TO BAKE A KID

Take your kid and parboil him, and wash it in verjuice and saffron, and season it with pepper, salt and a little mace.

Then lay it in your coffin with sweet butter and the liquor it was seasoned in. And so bake it.

TO BAKE A MALLARD

Take three or four onions and stamp them in a mortar. Then strain them in a saucer full of verjuice. Take your mallard and put him into the juice of the said onions, and season him with pepper and salt, cloves and mace. Then put your mallard into your coffin with the said juice of the onions and a good quantity of winter savory, a little thyme and parsley chopped small, and sweet butter. So close it up and bake it.

TO BAKE A RED DEER

Take a handful of thyme, a handful of rosemary, a handful of winter savory, a handful of bay leaves and a handful of fennel. When your liquor seethe that you parboil your venison in, put in your herbs also, and parboil your venison until it be half enough. Then take it out and lay it upon a fair board that the water may run out from it. Then take a knife and prick it full of holes. While it is warm have a fair tray with vinegar therein and so put your venison in from morning until night, and ever now and then turn it upside down. Then at night have your coffin ready. This done, season it with cinnamon, ginger, and nutmegs, pepper and salt. And when you have seasoned it, put it in your coffin and put a good quantity of sweet butter into it. Then put it into the oven at night when you go to bed. In the morning draw it forth and put a saucer full of vinegar into your pie at a hole in the top of it, so that the vinegar may run into every place of it. Then close up the hole again and turn the bottom upward. And so serve it in.

ANOTHER BAKE MEAT FOR CHICKENS

First season your chickens with sugar, cinnamon and ginger, and lay them in your pie. Then put in upon them gooseberries, or grapes, or barberries. Then put in some sweet butter and close them up. When they be almost baked, then put in a caudle made of hard eggs and white wine. And so serve it.

TO BAKE CALVE'S FEET

Take calve's feet and boil them and chop them fine. And a pound of white and chop it with them. Then chop an onion small and put it in them. Take prunes, dates and currants, and put to them. Season them with pepper, nutmegs, and a little large mace. Then put in some eggs and stir it altogether and put it into a pie. Let it bake two hours. Then put in a little verjuice and sugar. And so serve it.

FOR TO BAKE A HARE

Take your hare and parboil him and mince him, and then beat him in a mortar very fine, liver and all if you will. Season it with all kinds of spices and salt. Do him together with the yolks of seven or eight eggs. When you have made him up together, draw lard, very thick, through him, and mingle them altogether. Put him in a pie, and put in butter before you close him up.

TO BAKE THE HUMBLES OF A DEER

Mince them very small and season them with pepper, cinnamon and ginger, and sugar if you will, and cloves, mace, dates, and currants and, if you will, mince almonds, and put unto them. When it is baked you must put in fine fat, and sugar, cinnamon and ginger and let it boil. When it is minced put them together.

TO BAKE CALVE'S FEET

Season them with salt and pepper, and butter and currants if you will. When they be baked put in a little white wine and sugar, or vinegar and sugar, or verjuice and sugar.

TO BAKE CHICKENS IN A CAUDLE

Season them with salt and pepper and put in butter. And so let them bake. When they be baked boil a few barberries and prunes and currants, and take a little white wine or verjuice, and let it boil. Put in a little sugar, and set it on the fire a little, and strain in two or three yolks of eggs into the wine. When you take the dish off the fire put the prunes, currants and barberries into the dish. And then put them in altogether into the pie of chickens.

TO BAKE PIGEONS

Season them with pepper and salt and butter.

TO BAKE A CONEY

Season him with pepper and salt and put in butter and currants. When it is baked put in a little verjuice and sugar into the pie. And so serve it up.

TO BAKE A GAMMON OF BACON
TO KEEP COLD

You must first boil him a quarter of an hour before you

stuff him. Stuff him with sweet herbs and hard eggs, chopped together, or parsley.

TO BAKE A FILLET OF BEEF TO KEEP COLD

Mince him very small, and seethe him with pepper and salt, and make him up together accordingly, and put them in your pie. Lard him very thick.

TO BAKE A NEAT'S TONGUE

First ponder the tongue three or four days and seethe it in fair water. Then blanch it and lard it and season it with a little pepper and salt. Then bake it on rye paste. Before you close up your pie throw upon the tongue a good quantity of cloves and mace beaten in powder, and upon that half a pound of butter. Then close up your pie very close but make a round hole in the top of the pie. Then when it hath stood more than four hours in the oven, you must put in half a pint of vinegar or more, as vinegar is sharp. Then close up the hole very close with a piece of paste and set it in the oven again.

TO BAKE A HARE

Take your hare and parboil him, and mince him, and then beat him in a mortar very fine, liver and all if you will. And season him with all kinds of spice and salt, and do him together with the yolks of seven or eight eggs. When you have made him up together, draw lard , very thick, through him, or cut the lard and mingle them together, and put him in a pie and put in butter before you close him up.

TO BAKE ALOES OF VEAL OR MUTTON

Make your aloes ready to bake in all points as you boil them, laying upon them, in the paste, barberries, gooseberries, grapes green, or small raisins. Put in your pie a dish of butter. And so set it in the oven; and when it is baked, then put in a little verjuice, and so seethe it in an oven again a while. And so serve it forth.

TO BAKE A CONEY, VEAL, OR MUTTON

Take a conie and parboil it almost enough. Then mince the flesh of it very fine, and take with it three yolks of hard eggs and mince with it. Then lay another conie in your pie, being parboiled, and your minced meat with it, being seasoned with cloves, mace,ginger,saffron, pepper and salt, with two dishes of sweet butter mixed with it. Lay upon your conie barberries, gooseberries, grapes, or else small raisins. And so bake it.

TO BAKE A PORPOISE OR SEAL

Take your porpoise or seal, and parboil it, seasoning it with pepper and salt; and so bake it. You must take off the skin when you do bake it, and then serve it forth with galantine in saucers.

A TROUT BAKED OR MINCED

Take a trout and seethe him. Then take out all the bones. Then mince it very fine with three or four dates minced with it; seasoning it with ginger, and cinnamon, and a quantity of sugar and butter. Put all these together, working them fast. Then take your fine paste and cut it in three corner ways in a small bigness, of four or five coffins in a dish. Then lay your stuff in them, close them, and so bake them. And in the serving of them baste the covers with a little butter, and then cast a little blanch powder on them, and so serve it forth.

TO BAKE LAMPREYS

First make your coffin long ways. Season your Lampreys with pepper, cloves and mace, and put them in the pie. Put thereto a good handful of small raisins, two or three onions sliced, a good piece of butter, a little sugar, and a few barberries. When it is enough, put in a little verjuice.

TO BAKE CHICKENS

First season them with cloves, mace, pepper, and salt, and put to them currants and barberries. Slit an apple and cast cinnamon and sugar upon the apple, and lay it in the bottom. To it put a dish of butter, and when it is almost enough baked put a little sugar, verjuice, and oranges.

TO MAKE A PIE

First parboil your flesh and press it. And when it is pressed season it with pepper and salt whilst it is still hot. Then lard it. Make your paste with rye flour, it must be very thick or else it will not hold. And when it is seasoned and larded lay it in your pie. Then cast on it before you close it a good deal of cloves and mace, beaten small, and throw upon that a good deal of butter, and so close it up. You must leave a hole in the top of the lid, and when it hath stood two hours in the oven you must fill it as full of wine vinegar as you can. Then stop the hole as close as you can with oaste, and then set it into your oven again. Your oven must be very hot as the first, that your pies will keep a great while, the longer you keep them [in the oven] the better they will be. When they be taken out of the oven and almost cold you must shake them between you hands and set them with the bottom upward. When you set them into the oven be well ware that one pie touches not an other by more than a hands breadth. Remember also to let them stand in the oven after the vinegar be in two hours and more.

TO MAKE MARROW PIES

Make fine paste and put in the white of one egg and sugar. When they are made in little coffins set them into the oven upon a paper a little while. Then take them out and put in marrow, and then close them up and prick them, and set them in again. And when they are broken serve them with blanch ponder* strewed upon them.

* *White powder, probably powdered spices.*

FOR TO MAKE MUTTON PIES

Mince your mutton and your white together. When it is minced season it with pepper, cinnamon, ginger, cloves, mace, prunes, currants, dates and raisins, and hard eggs, boiled and chopped very small, and throw them on top.

TO MAKE A VEAL PIE

Let your veal boil a good while. When it is boiled mince it by itself, and the white by itself. Season it with salt and pepper, cinnamon and ginger, sugar cloves and mace. You must have prunes and raisins, dates and currants, on the top.

TO MAKE A PIE OF HUMBLES*

Take your humbles being parboiled, and chop them very small with a good quantity of mutton suet and half a handful

* *Innards.*

of herbs following: thyme, marjoram, borage, parsley, and a
little rosemary, and season the same, being chopped, with
pepper, cloves and mace. And so close your pie and bake
him.

TO MAKE OYSTER CHEWETS*

Take a peck of oysters and wash them clean, then shell
them and wash them fair in a collander, and when they be
sodden, strain the water from them, and chop them as small
as pie meat. Then season them with pepper, half a
pennyworth of cloves and mace, half a pennyworth of
cinnamon and ginger, and a pennyworth of sugar, a little
saffron and salt. Then take a handful of small raisins, six
dates, minced small, and mingle them altogether. Then make
your paste with one pennyworth of fine flour, ten yolks of
eggs, a halfpennyworth of butter with a little saffron, and
boiling water. Then raise up your chewets and put in the
bottom of every one of them a little butter. And so fill them
with your stuff. Then cast prunes, dates, and small raisins
upon them and, being closed, bake them. Let not your oven
be too hot for they will have but little baking. Then draw
them and put into every one two spoonfuls of verjuice and
butter. And so serve them.

* *Small pies.*

TO MAKE A PIE IN A POT

Take the leanest of a leg of mutton and mince it small,
with a piece of the kidney of mutton. Then put it into an
earthen pot, putting thereto a ladleful or two of mutton
broth, and a little wine, prunes and raisins, of each a handful,
or barberries.   Let them boil together, putting to it half an

orange, if you have any, seasoning it with salt, pepper, cloves, mace, and saffron, and so serve it.

TO MAKE FINE PASTE

Take fair flour and wheat and the yolks of eggs with sweet butter, melted; mixing all these together with your hands, till it be brought down paste. Then make your coffins, whether it be for pies or tarts. Then you may put saffron and sugar if you will have it a sweet paste. Having respect to the true seasoning some use to put to their paste beef or mutton broth, and some cream.

FOR SMALL PIES

Take the marrow out of the marrow bones whole, and cut it in the bigness of a bean. Season your marrow with ginger, and sugar, and cinnamon. Then put them in fine paste and fry them in a frying pan with the skimming of fresh beef broth, or else you may bake them in your oven a little while. Take heed they burn not. And when you do serve them in a fair dish, cast blanch powder upon them.

TO MAKE PURSES OR CREMITARIES*

Take a little marrow, small raisins, and dates, (let the stones be taken away) these being beaten together in a mortar. Season it with ginger, cinnamon, and sugar. Put it in fine paste and bake them or fry them. So done, in the serving of them cast blanch powder upon them.
* *Turnovers.*

TO MAKE A TART OF AN EAR OF VEAL

Take two pounds of great raisins, and wash them clean, and pick them, and take out the stones of them. Take two kidneys of veal, and a piece of the leg, which is lean. And boil them altogether in a pot with the strained broth of mutton. And boil it, and let it boil the space of one hour. Then take it up and chop it fine, and temper it with crumbs of bread, finely grated. Take nine yolks of eggs and temper them altogether. And season them with cinnamon, ginger, sugar, and small raisins, great raisins minced, dates and saffron. Then take fine flour and water, and three yolks of eggs, butter, saffron, and make them like a round tart, close with a cover of the same paste. Set him in the oven, and let him stand one hour. Then take him forth and adorn it with butter and cast a powder of cinnamon, ginger. and sugar, and so serve it.

TO MAKE BUTTER PASTE

Take flour and seven or eight eggs, and cold butter and fair water, or rose water, and spices (if you will) and make your paste . Beat it on a board, and when you have so done divide it into two or three parts and drive out the piece with a rolling pin. And do[t] with butter one piece by another, and fold up your paste upon the butter and drive it out again. And so do five or six times together, and some not cut for bearings. Put them into the oven, and when they be baked scrape sugar on them and serve them.

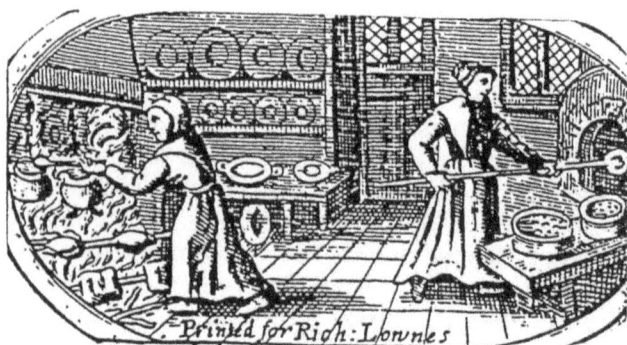

TO MAKE ALL MANNER OF FRUIT TARTS

You must boil your fruit whether it be apple, cherry, peaches, damson, pear, mulberry, or codling, in fair water. When they be boiled enough, put them into a bowl and bruise them with a ladle. When they be cold, strain them, and put in red wine, or claret wine, and so season it with sugar, cinnamon, and ginger.

TO BAKE A CITRON PIE

Take your citron, pare it and slice it in pieces. Boil it with gross pepper and ginger, and so lay it in your paste with butter. When it is almost baked, put thereto vinegar, butter, and sugar, and let it stand in the oven a while and soak.

ANOTHER WAY TO BAKE CITRONS

When your citrons be pared and sliced, lay it in your paste with small raisins, and season them with pepper, ginger, and fine sugar.

TO MAKE A TART OF PRESERVED STUFF

You must take half a hundred of costards* and pare them and cut them. As soon as you have cut them put them in a pot. Put in two or three pounds of sugar, and a pint of water, and a little rose water, and stir them from the time you put them in until the time you take them out again. Or else you may also put it into a dish. And when your tart is made, put it into the oven. When it is caked adorn it with butter, and throw sugar on the top. Then do your sauce, and set comfits on the top; and so serve it up.

* *Apples.*

TO MAKE A TART OF PRUNES

Put your prunes into a pot and put in red wine or claret wine, and a little fair water. Stir them now and then, and when they be boiled enough, put them into a bowl. Strain them with sugar, cinnamon and ginger.

TO MAKE A TART OF RICE

Boil your rice and put in the yolks of two or three eggs into the rice. When it is boiled, put it into a dish and season it with sugar, cinnamon and ginger, and butter, and the juice of two or three oranges, and set it on the fire again.

TO MAKE A TART OF WARDENS*

You must bake your wardens first in a pie. Then take all the wardens and cut them in four quarters, and core them and put them into a tart, pinched, with your sugar. Season them with sugar, cinnamon and ginger, and set them in the oven. Put no cover on them but you must cut a cover and lay

it on the tart when it is baked. Butter the tart and the cover too, and adorn it with sugar.
* *Warden pears.*

TO MAKE A TART WITH BUTTER AND EGGS

Break your eggs and take the yolks of them. And take butter and melt it. Let it be very hot, ready to boil. Put your butter into your eggs and so strain them into a bowl and season them with sugar.

TO MAKE A TART OF STRAWBERRIES

Wash your strawberries and put them into your tart. Season them with sugar, cinnamon and ginger, and put a little red wine into them.

TO MAKE A TART OF HIPS

Take hips and cut them and take the seeds out. Wash them very clean and put them into your tart. Season them with sugar, cinnamon and ginger. So you must preserve them with sugar, cinnamon and ginger, and put them into a gally pot*, close.
* *A small earthen pot, usually glazed.*

FOR TARTS OF CREAM

Take a pint of cream with six raw eggs, and boil them together. Stir it well that it burn not and then let it boil till it be thick. Then take it out of the pot and put to two dishes of butter, melted. When it is somewhat cold, then strain it and season it with sugar. Then put it into your paste. When your paste is hardened, and when it is enough, then serve it with sugar cast upon it. If you will have a tart of two colours, then take the half of it, when it is in cream, and colour the other half with saffron or yolks of eggs.

A TART OF PROINES*

Make your coffin two inches deep round about. Then take ten or twelve good apples, pare them and slice them, and put them into the paste with two dishes of butter among the apples. Then cover your tart close with the paste, and break a dish of butter in pieces, and lay it upon the cover because of burning in the pan. And when the apples be tender take it forth and cut off the cover, and beat the apples together till they be soft. And [if] they be dry put more butter into them. And so season them with cinnamon, ginger, and sugar. Then must you cut your cover after the fashion, leaving it upon your tarts. Serve it with blanch powder.
* *Prunes. A mistaken title for this apple recipe.*

TO MAKE A TART OF SPINACH

Boil your eggs and your cream together and then put them into a bowl. Then boil your spinach, and when they are boiled take them out of the water and strain them into your stuff before you strain your cream. Boil your stuff and then strain them all again. Season them with sugar and salt.

TO MAKE A TART OF SPINACH

Take spinach and seethe it stalk and all. And when it is tenderly sodden, take it off, and let it drain in a collander. Then let it swing in a cloth, and stamp it and strain it with two or three yolks of eggs. Then set it on a chafing dish of coals, and season it with butter and sugar. And when the

paste is hardened in the oven, put in this comode,* [and] stroke it even.
* *Mixture.*

TO MAKE A CLOSE TART OF GREEN PEAS

Take half a peck of green peas, sheal* them and seethe them, and cast them into a collander, and let the water go from them. Then put them into a tart whole. Season them with pepper, saffron, and salt, and a dish of sweet butter. Close and bake him almost one hour. Then draw him and put to him a little verjuice, and shake them and let them into the oven again, and so serve it.
* *Shell.*

TO MAKE A TART OF SPINACH OR OF WHEAT LEAVES OR OF COLEWORTS

Take three handfuls of spinach; boil it in fair water. When it is boiled, put away the water from it and put the spinach in a stone mortar; grind it small with two dishes of butter, melted, and four raw eggs, all to [be] beaten. Then strain it and season it with sugar, cinnamon, and ginger, and lay it in your coffin. When it is hardened in the oven, then bake it. When it is enough serve it upon a fair dish, and cast upon it sugar and biscuits.

A TART OF EGGS

Take twelve eggs and butter them together. Then strain them with rose water; season it with sugar. Then put it into your paste. And so bake it and serve it with sugar upon it.

TO MAKE A TART OF STRAWBERRIES

Take strawberries and wash them in claret wine, thicken and temper them with rose water, and season them with cinnamon, sugar and ginger, and spread it on the tart. And adorn the sides with butter and cast on sugar and biscuits and serve them so.

TO MAKE A CLOSE TART OF CHERRIES

Take out the stones, and lay them as whole as you can in a charger. And put mustard in cinnamon and ginger to them, and lay them in a tart whole, and close them. Let them stand three quarters of an hour in the oven. Then take a syrup of muscadine, and damask water and sugar, and serve it.

TO MAKE A TART OF DAMSONS

Take damsons and seethe them in wine. Strain them with a little cream. Then boil your stuff over the fire till it be thick. Put thereto sugar, cinnamon, and ginger, but let it not into the oven after, but let your paste be baked before.

TO MAKE A TART OF MEDLARS

Take medlars that be rotten and stamp them. Then set them on a chafing dish with coals, and beat in two yolks of eggs, boiling it till it be somewhat thick. Then season them with sugar, cinnamon and ginger and lay it in the paste.

TO MAKE TARTS OR BALDE* MEATS
FOR FISH DAYS

Take your dish and annoint the bottom well with butter. Then make a fine paste to the breadth of the dish, and lay it on the same dish upon the butter. Then take beets, spinach, and cabbages or white lettuce, cutting them fine, in long pieces. Then take the yolks of eight raw eggs, and six yolks of hard eggs, with small raisins and a little cheese fine scraped, and grated bread, and three or four dishes of butter, melted and clarified. And when you have wrought it together, season it with sugar, cinnamon, ginger, and salt. Then lay it upon your fine paste, spreading it abroad: then the cover of fine paste being cut with pretty work. Then set it in your oven [and] bake it with your dish under it. When it is enough, then at the serving of it you must new paste the cover of it with butter, scrape sugar upon it, and so serve it forth.

* *Leaf.*

TO MAKE FINE CRACKNELS

Take fine flour and a good quantity of eggs, as many as will supply the flour. Then take as much sugar as will sweeten the paste. If you will not be at the cost to raise it with eggs, put thereto sweet water, cinnamon and a good quantity of nutmegs and mace. According to your bread take a good quantity of aniseed and let all this be blended with your flour and the putting in of your eggs or other moisture. Then set on your water and let it be at seething before you put your cracknels in it. They will go to the bottom, and at their rising take them out and dry them with a cloth. Then bake them.

TO MAKE FINE BISCUIT BREAD

Take a pound of fine flour, and a pound of sugar, and mingle it together [with] a quarter of a pound of aniseeds, four eggs, [and] two or three spoonfuls of rose water. Put all these into an earthen pan and with a slice of wood beat it the space of two hours. Then fill your moulds half full. Your moulds must be of tin. Then let it into your oven, being so hot as it were for cheat* bread. Let it stand one hour and an half. You must anoint your moulds with butter before you put in your stuff. And when you will occupte** of it, slice it thin and dry it in your oven, your oven being no hotter than you may abide your hand in the bottom.

* *Second quality coarse bread, usually dark.*
** *Make use of.*

TO MAKE FINE BREAD

Take half a pound of fine sugar, well beaten, and as much flour, and put thereto four egg whites, being very well beaten. You must mingle them with aniseeds, bruised, and being all beaten together put into your mould, melting the sauce over first with a little butter. Set it in the oven and turn it twice or thrice in the baking.

TO MAKE BISCUIT BREAD

First take half a peck of fine white flour, also eight new laid eggs, the whites and yolks beaten together. Then put the said eggs into the flour. Then take eight grains of fine musk and stamp it in a mortar. Then put half a pint of good damask water, or else rose water, into the musk, and mingle it together and put it into wine or muscadine, but muscadine is better. Put it into the flour, also one ounce of good aniseeds, clean picked and put therein. And so to work them altogether into a paste, as ye do bread. Then make your biscuits into what fashion you think best. Then put them into an oven and bake them hard , if you will keep them long, or else but indifferent. If you will have it candied, take rose water and sugar and boil them together till they be thick, and so slices of bread. Then set hot in the oven until the same be candied.

TO MAKE FINE CAKES

Take fine flour and damask water. You must have no other liquor but that. Then take sweet butter, two or three yolks of eggs and a good quantity of sugar,and a few cloves, and mace as your cook's mouth shall serve him, and a little saffron, and a little cods* good, about a spoonful. If you put in too much they shall arise. Cut them in squares like unto trenchers and prick them well. Let your oven be well swept. Lay them upon papers and so set them in the oven. Do not burn them. If they be three or four days old they be the better.

Balm, yeast.

TO MAKE MANUS CHRISTI*

Take five spoonfuls of rose water, and grains of ambergrease,** and four grains of pearl, beaten very fine. Put these things together in a saucer and cover it close. Let it stand covered one hour. Then take four ounces of very fine sugar, and beat it small, and search*** it through a fine search. Then take a little earthen pot, glazed, and put into it a spoonful of sugar, and a quarter of a spoonful of rose water, and let the sugar and rose water boil together softly till it do rise and fall again three times. Then take fine rye flour and sift on a smooth board.   And with a spoon take of the

* *Hand of Christ.*
** *A secretion from the intestines of the sperm whale, much used in cookery at this time. Now used in perfumery.*
*** *Sieve.*

sugar and the rose water, and first make it all into a round cake and then into little cakes. When they be half cold, wet them over with some rose water, and then lay on your gold. And so shall you make very good Manus Christi.

TO MAKE JOMBILS,* A HUNDRED

Take twenty eggs and put them into a pot, both the yolks and the white; beat them well. Then take a pound of beaten sugar and put to them, and stir them well together. Then put to it a quarter of a peck of flour and make a hard paste thereof; and then with aniseed mould it well and make it in little rolls, being long. Tie them in knots, and wet the ends in rose water. Then put them into a pan of seething water, but even in one waum. Then take them out with a skimmer and lay them in a cloth to dry. This being done, lay them in a tart pan, the bottom being oiled. Then put them into a temperate oven for one hour, turning them often in the oven.
* *Jumbles.*

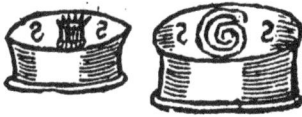

The Forms of double bordered Cultards

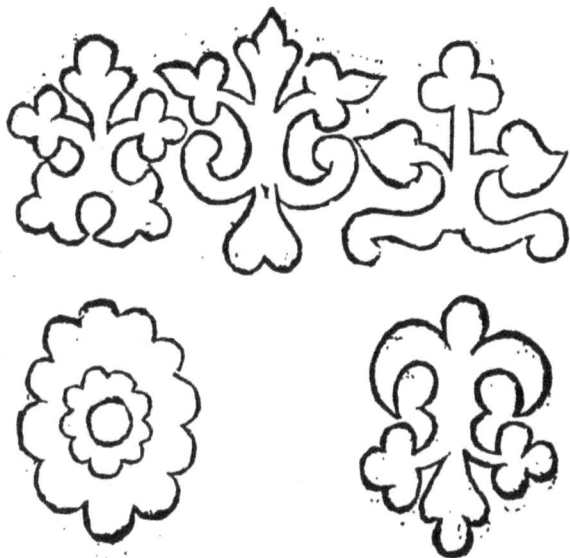

EGGS

CREAM

TO MAKE BUTTERED EGGS

Take eight yolks of eggs and put them into a pint of cream. Beat them together and strain them all into a posnet, setting upon the fire and stirring it. Let it seethe until it quaile,* then take it and put it into a clean cloth, and let it hang so that the whey may void from it. When it is gone, beat it into a dish of rosewater and sugar with a spoon. So shall you have fine butter. This done, you may take the white of the same eggs, putting it into another pint of cream, using it as the yolks were used. And thus you may have as fine white butter as you have yellow butter.

* *Curdle.*

TO MAKE A CUSTARD

Break your eggs into a bowl, and put your cream into another bowl. Strain your eggs into the cream. Put in saffron, cloves and mace, and a little cinnamon and ginger, and, if you will, some sugar and butter. Season it with salt. Melt your butter and stir it with the ladle a good while. Dub your custard with dates or currants.

TO MAKE BLEWMANGER

Take to a pint of cream, twelve or thirteen yolks of eggs, and strain them into it. And seethe them well, ever stirring it with a stick that is broad at the end. But before you seethe it put in sugar and in the seething taste of it,that you may, if need be, put in more sugar. And when it is almost sodden put in a little rose water that it may taste thereof. Seethe it well till it be thick, and then strain it again if it hath need, or else put it into a fair dish and stir it till it be almost cold. Take the white of all the eggs and strain them with a pint of cream and seethe that with sugar, and in the end put in rose water as into the other, and seethe till it be thick enough.

Then use it as the other. When you serve it you may serve one dish, and another of the other in rolls, and cast on biscuits.

TO MAKE GOOD RESBONES*

Take a quart of fine flour, lay it upon a fair board and make a hole in the middle of the flour with your hand, and put a spoonful of ale yeast thereon, and ten yolks of eggs and two spoonfuls of cinnamon, one of ginger,and one of cloves and mace, and a quarterne of sugar finely beaten, and a little saffron and half a spoon of salt. Then take a dish full of butter, melt it and put it into your flour and there withal make your paste as it were for manchet. Mould it a good while and cut it in pieces of the bigness of ducks eggs, and so mould every piece as a manchet. Make them after the fashion of an inkhorn, broad above and narrow beneath. Then let them bake three quarters of an hour. Then take two dishes of butter and clarify it upon a soft fire. Draw it out of the oven, and scrape the bottom of them fair and clean, and cut them overthwart in four pieces, and put them in a fair charger. Put your clarified butter upon them, and have cinnamon and ginger ready by you, and sugar beaten small, and mingle together. And ever as you set your pieces together, cast some of your sugar, cinnamon and ginger upon them. When you have set them all up, lay them in a fair platter and put a little butter upon them and cast a little sugar on them. And so serve them.

* *Cheesecake.*

TO FARCE EGGS

Take eight or ten eggs and boil them hard.Peel off the shells and cut every egg in the middle; then take out the yolks. Make your farcing stuff as you do for flesh, saving only you must put butter into it instead of suet, and that a little. So done, fill your eggs where the yolks were, and then bind them them and seethe them a little. And so serve them to the table.

TO MAKE A LENTEN HAGGIS WITH
POACHED EGGS

Take a skillet of a pint, and fill it half with verjuice and half with water. Then take marjoram, winter savory, pennyroyal, mints, thyme, of each six crops. Wash them, and take four eggs, hard roasted, and shred them as fine as you can. Put the herbs thus into the broth. Then put a great handful of currants, and the crumbs of a quarter of a manchet, and so let it seethe till it be thick. Then season it with sugar, cinnamon, salt and a good piece of butter, and three or four spoonfuls of rose water. Then poach seven eggs and lay them on sippets. Pour the haggis on them, with cinnamon and sugar strewed on them.

TO MAKE ALMOND CUSTARD

Take a good sort of almonds, blanched. Stamp them with water, and strain them with water and a little rose water and twelve eggs. Then season it with a little cinnamon, sugar, and a good deal of ginger. Then set it upon a pot of seething water. When it is enough stick dates in it.

TO MAKE ALMOND BUTTER AFTER THE BEST
AND NEWEST FASHION

Take a pound of almonds or more, and blanch them in cold water or in warm as you may have leisure. After the blanching let them lie one hour in cold water. Then stamp them in fair cold water as fine as you can. Then put your almonds in a cloth, and gather your cloth round up in your hands, and press out the juice as much as you can. If you think they be not small enough, beat them again. And so get out milk so long as you can. Then set it over the fire, and when it is ready to seethe, put in a good quantity of salt, and rose water that will turn it. After that is in, let it have one boiling. Then take it from the fire and cast it abroad upon a linen cloth and underneath the cloth scrape off the whey so long as it will run. Then put the butter together into the middle of the cloth, binding the cloth together, and let it hang so long as it will drop. Then take pieces of sugar, so much as you think will make it sweet, and put thereto a little rose water, so much as will melt the sugar, and so much fine powder of saffron as you think will colour it. Then let both your sugar and saffron steep together in the little quantity of rose water. And with that season up your butter when you will make it.

TO MAKE FRESH CHEESE AND CREAM

Take a gallon of milk from the cow, and seethe it, and when it doth seethe put thereunto a quart or two of morning milk in fair cleansing pans, in such place as no dust may fall therein. This is for your clotted cream. The next morning take a quart of morning milk, and seethe it, and put in a quart of cream thereunto, and when it doth seethe, take it off the fire. Put it in a fair earthen pan, and let it stand until it be somewhat blood warm. But first over night put a good quantity of ginger, with rose water, and stir it together. Let it settle all night. The next day put it into your said bloodwarm milk to make your cheese come. Then put the curds in a fair cloth, with a little good rose water, fine powder of ginger, and a little sugar. So lash great soft rolls together with a thread and crush out the whey with your clotted cream. Mix it with fine powder of ginger, and sugar, and so sprinkle it with rose water, and put your cheese in a fair dish. And put these clots round about it. Then take a pint of raw milk or cream and put it in a pot, and all to shake it until it be gathered into a froth like snow. And ever as it cometh, take it off with a spoon and put it into a collander. Then put it upon your fresh cheese, and prick it with wafers, and so serve it.

TO MAKE CAST CREAM

Take milk as it commeth from the cow, a quart or less, and put thereto raw yolks of eggs. Temper the milk and eggs together. Then set the same upon a chafing dish and stir it that it curd not. And so put a sugar in it, and it will be like cream of almonds. When it is boiled thick enough cast a little sugar on it and sprinkle rose water thereupon. And so serve it.

A WHITE LEACH

Take a quart of new milk and three ounces weight of isinglass,* half a pound of beaten sugar; stir them together. Let it boil half a quarter of an hour till it be thick, stirring them all the while. Then strain it with three spoonfuls of rose water. Then put it into a platter and let it cool, and cut it in squares. Lay it fair in dishes, and lay gold upon it.

A substance obtained from the swim bladders of freshwater fish, used as gelatin.

TO MAKE A BLANCH MANGER ON THE FIFTH DAY

Take whites of eggs and cream and boil them on a chafing dish on coals till they curd. Then will their whey go from them; then put away their whey. Then put to the curd a little rose water. Strain it and season it with sugar.

TO MAKE ICING PUDDINGS

Take great oatmeal and pick it and let it soak in thick cream three hours. Then put thereto yolks of eggs, and some whites, pepper, salt, cloves and mace, and a little sugar. Fill them not too full and seethe them a good while.

TO MAKE A TRIFLE

Take a pint of thick cream, and season it with sugar and ginger, and rose water. So stir it as you would then have it and make it luke warm in a dish on a chafing dish and coals. And after put it into a silver piece or a bowl, and so serve it to the board.

TO MAKE ALMOND BUTTER

Take almonds and blanch them and beat them in a mortar very small. In the beating put in a little water. When they be beaten pour in water into two pots, and put in one half into one and half into another. Put in sugar and stir them still and let them boil a good while. Then strain it through a strainer with rose water. And so dish it up.

FRUIT

PRESERVING

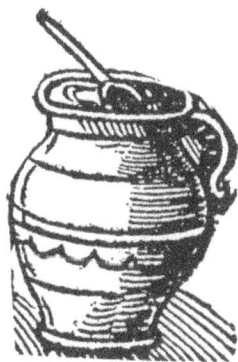

TO MAKE A QUINCES MOYSE* OR A
WARDENS MOYSE

You must roast your wardens or quinces, and when they be roasted peel them and strain them together. And put in sugar, cinnamon and ginger, and put it in a plate. Then smooth it with a knife and scrape a little sugar on the top, and nick a little with a knife.

* *Fruit moyse, or muse, a favourite of the fifteenth century.*

TO MAKE APPLE MOYSE

Roast your apples, and when they be roasted, peal them and strain them into a dish. Pare a dozen of apples and cut them into a chafer. Put in a little white wine and a little butter and let them boil till they be as soft as pap. Stir them a little, and strain them to some wardens, roasted and pealed, and put in sugar, cinnamon and ginger. Make diamonds of the paste, and lay them in the sun. Then scrape a little sugar upon them in the dish.

TO BAKE QUINCES, PEARS, AND WARDENS

Take and pare and core them. Then make your paste with fair water and butter, and the yolk of an egg. Then set the oranges into the paste and then bake it well. Fill your paste almost full with cinnamon, ginger and sugar. Also apples must be taken after the same sort, saving that whereas the core should be cut out, they must be filled with butter every one. The hardest apples are best, and likewise are pears and wardens, and none of them all but the wardens may be parboiled. The oven must be of a temperate heat. Two hours to stand is enough.

TO MAKE MELONS AND POMPONS* SWEET

Take fine sugar and dissolve it in water, then take seeds of melons and cleave them a little on the side that sticketh to the melon. Put them in the sugared water, adding to them a little rose water. Leave the said seeds so, by the space of three or four hours, then take them out, and you shall see that as soon as the said seeds be dry, it will close up again. Plant it, and there will come of it such melons as the like hath not been seen. If you will have them give the savour of musk, put in the said water a little musk and fine cinnamon. And thus you may do the seeds of pompons and cucumbers.
* *Large melon or pumpkin.*

TO MAKE ANOTHER PRETTY DISH WITH DATES AND THE JUICE OF TWO OR THREE ORANGES

Strain them into a dish. And so make chambers of paste upon a stick, put the sticks upon a loaf of bread. And so dry them in the oven. Then clarify a little butter and fry them in it, and lay them in a dish, and serve sugar on them.

TO MAKE MARMELET OF QUINCES

Take very good quinces and pare them and cut them in quarters. Then core them clean, and take heed it be not a stony quince. And when you have pared and cored them, then take two pints of running water and put it into a brass pan, casting away eight spoonfuls of one of the pints. Then weigh three pounds of fine sugar and beat it and put it into the water. Make your fire where you may have a good light, not in a chimney. Then set your pan upon a trivet, and when your sugar and water beginneth to boil you must skim it clean. Then put in six spoonfuls of rose water and if there rise any more scum take it off. And so put in your three pounds of quinces and let them boil but softly. If you see the colour were somewhat deep, now and then with a fair slice be breaking of them. When your liquor is well consumed away, and the colour of your quinces to grow fairer, then be still stirring of it. When it is enough you shall see it rising from the bottom of your pan in the stirring of it. And so box it, and you shall have it to be good marmelet and a very orient colour. If you will you may put some musk into it, some rose water, and rub your box withal. It will give it a pretty scent and it is a very good way.

TO MAKE A MARMELAT OF QUINCES

You must take a pottle of water, and four pounds of sugar, and so let them boil together. When they boil you must skim them as clean as you can. You must take the whites of two or three eggs and beat them to froth. Put the froth into the pan for to make the scum to rise. Then skim it as clean as you can and take off the kettle and put in the quinces. Let them boil a good while. And when they boil you must stir them still. When they be boiled you must bore them up.

TO PRESERVE ORANGES

You must cut your oranges in half and pare them a little round about. Let them lie in water four or five days. You must change the water once or twice a day. And when you preserve them you must have a quart of fair water to put in your sugar, and a little rose water. Set it on the fire and scum it very clean. Put in a little cinnamon and put in your oranges. Let them boil a lttle while and take them out again. Do so five or six times, and when they be enough, put in your oranges and let your syrup stand till it be cold. Then put your syrup into your oranges.

TO PRESERVE QUINCES WHOLE

Take a pottle of fair water and put it into a clean pan, and beat three pounds of fine sugar and put into it. Then set it on the fire, and when you have skimmed it, put in twelve spoonfuls of rose water. Then take five quinces and pare them and core them clean. Then put them into your syrup and cover them very close for the space of two hours with a fair platter. Let them boil at a good pace the two hours, and uncover them and look whether you find them tender and that they have a fair crimson colour. Then take them up, and lay them upon a fair platter, covering your syrup again. Let it seethe while it be somewhat thick. Put your quinces into your syrup again, and so have a fair gallypot and put both in your syrup and quinces as fast as you can and cover your pot close that the heat go not forth. You must not put them in a glass for it will break.

TO PRESERVE PEAR PLUMS

First take two pounds and a half of fine sugar and beat it small. Put it into a pretty brass pot with twenty spoonfuls of rose water, and when it boileth skim it clean. Then take it off the fire and let it stand while it be almost cold. Then take two pounds of pear plums, and wipe them upon a fair cloth, and put them into your syrup when it is almost cold. And so set them upon the fire again, and let them boil as softly as you can. When they are boiled enough the kernels will be yellow. Then take them up, but let your syrup boil till it be thick. Then put your plums upon the fire again and let them boil a walme* or two. So take them from the fire and let them stand in the vessel all night. In the morning put them into your pot or glass and cover them close.
* *A short period of boiling.*

TO PRESERVE ORANGES

Choose out the fairest and the heaviest that is full of
liquor and cut them full of little specks. Then make a little
round hole in the stalks of the oranges, and break the strings
of the meat of the oranges, and close the meat to the sides of
your oranges with your finger. Then will part of the juice and
the kernels come out. Lay them in water three days and three
nights. Then take them out and set a pan with water over the
fire and when it seethes put in your oranges. Let them not
seethe too fast. Then you must have another pan with water
ready seething to shift your oranges out of the other water
when they have sodden a pretty while. And so have one pan
after another to shift them still upon the fire ten or twelve
times, to take away the bitterness of the oranges. You must
keep them as whole as you can in the boiling. Then take
them up one by one and lay them upon a platter, the hole
downward, that the water may run the clearer out of them. ·
Then let them stand so until you have boiled your syrup
ready for them. Now to make your syrup: take to every two
oranges a pint of water, and a pound of sugar. Let your sugar
be finely beaten before you put it into your liquor and look
that the kettle you boil them in be sweet brass. Then take ten
whites of eggs and put them into your kettle with your liquor
and sugar, and beat your whites of eggs and the liquor
together a good quarter of an hour. Set your liquor upon a
soft fire of coals and let it seethe so soon as you can, having
a fair skimmer and a collander ready. And set your collander
in a fair basin, and as your whites of eggs riseth in scum take
them up with your skimmer and put them in your collander.
You shall have a great quantity of syrup come from your
scum through your collander into your basin, and that you
must save and put it into your kettle again. When your scum
is off there will arise still some scum which you must take off
with a skimmer, as clean as you can. When your syrup hath
sodden a pretty while, then put in your oranges, and let them
boil softly, till you think they be enough. The syrup must be

somewhat thick. Then let your oranges stand all night upon the fire, but there must be nothing but embers. In the morning take them up and put them in glasses or gallypots.

TO PRESERVE QUINCES IN SYRUP ALL THE YEAR

Take three pounds of quinces, being pared and cored, two pounds of sugar and three quarts of fair running water. Put all these together in an earthen pan, and let them boil with a soft fire. When they be skimmed, cover them close that no air may come out from them. You must put cloves and cinnamon to it after it is skimmed, of quantity as you will have them to taste. If you will know when they be boiled enough, hang a linen cloth between the cover and the pan, so that a good deal of it may hang in the liquor. When the cloth is very red, they be boiled enough. Let them stand till they be cold. Then put them in gally pots [with] syrup, and so they will keep a year.

TO CONSERVE WARDENS ALL THE YEAR
IN SYRUP

Take your wardens and put them into a great earthen pot, and cover them close. Set them in an oven when you have set in your white bread. When you have drawn your white bread and your pot, and that they be so cold that you can handle them, then peel the skins from them over a pewter dish, that you may save all the syrup that falleth from them. Put to them a quart of the same syrup, and a pint of rose water, and boil them together with a few cloves and cinnamon. When it is reasonably thick and cold, put your wardens and syrup into a gally pot. See always that the syrup be above the wardens, or any other thing that you conserve.

TO CONFIT WALNUTS

Take them green and small in husk, and make in them four little holes, or more, then steep them in water eleven days. Make them clean and boil them as the oranges hereafter written, but they must seethe four times as much. Dress them likewise with spices, saving you must put in very few cloves lest they taste bitter. In like sort you may dress gourds, cutting them in long pieces, and paring away the inner parts.

TO CONFIT ORANGE PEELS, WHICH MAY BE DONE AT ALL TIMES IN THE YEAR AND CHIEFLY IN MAY, BECAUSE THEN THE SAID PEELS BE GREATEST AND THICKEST

Take thick orange peels and then cut them in four or five pieces and steep them in water the space of ten or twelve days. You may know when they be steeped enough, if you hold them up in the sun and see through them, then they be steeped enough. If you cannot see through them, then let them steep until you may. Then lay them to dry upon a table, and put them to dry between two linen cloths. Then put them in a a kettle, or vessel leaded, and add to it as much honey as will half cover the said peels, more or less as you think good. Boil them a little and stir them always,then take them from the fire lest the honey should seethe over much. For if it should boil a little more than it ought to boil it would be thick. Let it stand and rest four days in the said honey, stirring and mingling the orange and honey every day together.Because there is not honey enough to cover all the said orange peels you must stir them well and oftentimes. Thus do three times, giving them one boiling at each time, then let them stand three days. Then strain them from the honey, and after you have let them boil a short space, then take them from the fire, and bestrew them in vessels; putting to them ginger,cloves,and cinnamon. Mix all together, and the rest of the syrup will serve to dress others withal.

TO CONSERVE CHERRIES, DAMSONS, OR WHITE PLUMS, ALL THE YEAR IN THE SYRUP

First take fair water, so much as you shall think meet, and one pound of sugar, and put them both into a fair basin. Set the same over a soft fire till the sugar be melted. Then put thereto one pound and a half of cherries, or damsons, and let them boil till they break. Then cover them close till they be cold. Then put them in your gally pots, and so keep them.This wise keeping proportion in weight of sugar and fruit you may conserve as much as you list, putting thereto cinnamon and cloves as is aforesaid.

TO MAKE CONDOMACKE OF QUINCES

Take five quarts of running water and a quart of French wine, put them together, and then take quinces and pare them and cut them till you come at the cores. Then weigh ten pounds of the quinces and put them into your pan of water and wine and boil them over a quick fire till they be tender, keeping your pan very close covered. Then take a piece of fine canvas and put your quinces and liquor in it. And when your syrup is all run through put in so much fine sugar as will make it sweet. And set it over a quick fire again, stirring with a stick till it be so thick that a drop will stand upon a dish. Then take it from the fire and put it in boxes.

TO MAKE A CONDOMACK

Take quinces and pare them. Take out the cores and seethe them in fair water until they break. Then strain them through a fine strainer, and for eight pounds of the said strained quinces you must put in three pounds of sugar, and mingle it together in a vessel. Boil them on the fire, always stirring it until it be sodden, which you may perceive, for that it will no longer cleave to the vessel. But you may stamp musk in powder, you may also add spice to it, as ginger, cinnamon, cloves, and nutmegs, as much as you think meet, boiling the musk with a little vinegar. Then with a broad slice of wood spread of this confection upon a table, which must be first strewed with sugar. And there make what proportion you will, and set it in the sun until it be dry. When it hath stood a while, turn it upside down, making always a bed of sugar, both under and above. Turn them still, and dry them in the sun until they have gotten a crust. In like manner you may dress pears, peaches, damsons, and other fruits.

TO MAKE SYRUP OF VIOLETS

First gather a great quantity of violet flowers, and pick them clean from the stalks. Set them on the fire and put to them so much rose water as you think good. Then let them boil altogether until the colour be forth of them. Then take them off the fire and strain them through a fine cloth. Then put so much sugar to them as you think good. Then set it again to the fire until it be somewhat thick. Put it into a viol glass.*
* *Glass phial.*

TO PRESERVE ORANGES

Take your peels and water them two nights and one day. Dry them clean again and boil them with a soft fire the space of one hour. Then take them out to cool. Make your syrup half with rosewater and half with that liquor, and put double sugar to your oranges. When your syrup is half sodden, then let your oranges seethe one quarter of an hour more. Then take out your oranges and let the syrup seethe until it rope.

When all is cold, then put your oranges into the syrup. The white of an egg and sugar beaten together will make it to candy.

TO MAKE DRY MARMELET OF PEACHES

Take your peaches and pare them and cut them from the stones, and mince them very finely. Steep them in rose water, then strain them with rose water through a coarse cloth or strainer, into your pan that you will seethe it in. You must have to every pound of peaches half a pound of sugar, finely beaten, and put it in your pan that you do boil it in. You must reserve out a good quantity to mould your cakes or prints withal, of that sugar. Set your pan on the fire and stir it till it be thick or stiff, that your stick will stand upright in it of itself. Then take it up and lay it in a platter or charger, in pretty lumps, as big as you will have the mould or prints. When it is cold print it on a fair board, with sugar; print them on a mould or whatnot, or fashion [as] you will. Bake in an earthen pot or pan upon the embers, or in a seat cover, and keep them continually by the fire to keep them dry.

TO MAKE THE SAME OF QUINCES
OR ANY OTHER THING

Take the quinces and quarter them and cut out the cores and pare them clean. Seethe them in fair water till they be very tender. Then take them with rose water and strain them, and do as is aforesaid in every thing.

TO PRESERVE ORANGES, LEMONS,
AND POMECITRONS*

First shave your oranges finely and put them into water two days and two nights, changing your water three times a day. Then parboil them in three several waters. Then take so much water as you think convenient for the quantity of your oranges. Then put in for every pound of oranges one pound and a half of sugar into the water, and put in two whites of eggs and beat them altogether. Then set them on the fire in a brass vessel, and when they boil skim them very clean, and cleanse them through a jelly bag. Then set it on the fire and put in the oranges. Use walnuts in like manner, and use lemons and pomecitrons in like sort, but they must lie in water but one night.

* A fruit larger than a lemon, thicker in rind and less acid.

TO PRESERVE QUINCES ALL YEAR THROUGH
WHOLE AND SOFT

Take, as is aforesaid, one pound of water and three pounds of sugar, and break it up into very small pieces, and do in all things as you did before. Then take twelve quinces and core them very clean, and pare them and wash them, and put [them] into your syrup. When the skim is taken off let them seethe until they be tender. Then take them up very soft for [fear of] breaking, and lay them in a fair thing, one by another. Then strain your syrup and set it on the fire again. Then put in your quinces and have a quick fire; let them seethe apace and turn them with your stick. When they be almost ready, put in some rose water and let them seethe. When you think they be ready, take up some of the syrup in a spoon, and if it be thick like a jelly when it is cold, then take of your pan and put your quinces into pots and your syrup to them. Put into your pots little sticks of cinnamon and a few cloves. When they be cold cover them with paper pricked full of small holes.

TO MAKE CONFECTIONS OF MELONS
OR POMPONES

Take what quantity of melons you think best and take them before they be ripe, but let them be good. Make as many cuts in them as they be marked with quarters on every side, and having mundified* them, and taken out the cores and kernels and peeled the outer rind, steep them in good vinegar, leaving them so the space of ten days. And when you have taken them out, take other vinegar and steep them anew again another ten days stirring them every day. Then when [the] time shall be, take them out, and put them in a coarse linen cloth, drying and wiping them, and set them in the air the space of a day and a night. Then boil them in honey, and by the space of ten days give them every day a little boiling, leaving them always in the honey. They must boil at every boiling but one walm. Then take the pieces and put them in a pot with powder of cloves, ginger, nutmegs, and pieces of cinnamon. Thus done, make one bed of the pieces of melon, and another of the spices, and then pour white honey upon all in the said pots or vessels.

* *Cleansed.*

TO MAKE QUINCES IN SYRUP

Take thirty quinces to the quantity of this syrup. Take a pottel of water and put it in a pan. Then take the whites of six eggs, and beat them with another pottel of water. Then put it altogether and put thereto twelve or fourteen pounds of sugar, as you shall see cause. Seethe and skim it very clean. Then put to it two ounces of cloves, and bruise them a very little and let them seethe until the same do rise very black. Then skim off the cloves again, and wash them in fair water, and dry them, and put them in again, and your quinces also. Put to them half a pint of rose water, and then put the syrup in a fair earthen pot, or pan, and lay a sheet four times double upon them to keep in the heat. So let it stand a day or two. Then put them and the syrup into a vessel that was never occupied and cover them close. But in the beginning pare your quinces and core them, and seethe them in fair water until they be tender. Then take them up and lay them that the water may run from them clean. When they be cold then put them into your syrup, as it is above said.

TO MAKE CONSERVE OF BARBERRIES

Take your barberries and pick them clean and set them over a soft fire, and put to them rose water as much as you think good. Then when you think it be sod enough, strain that, and then seethe it again. To every pound of barberries, one pound of sugar, and meat your conserve.

TO PRESERVE CHERRIES

To every pound of cherries take a pound of sugar. That done, take a few cherries and strain them to make your syrup, and to every pound, a pound of sugar and cherries. Take a quarter of a pound of syrup, and this done, take your syrup and sugar and set it on the fire. Then put your cherries into your syrup and let them boil five several times. After every boiling skim them with the backside of a spoon.

HOW TO PURIFY AND PREPARE HONEY
AND SUGAR
FOR TO CONFIT CITRONS AND ALL
OTHER FRUITS

Take every time ten pounds of honey, the whites of twelve new laid eggs, beat them well together with a stick and take away the froth of them, and six glasses of fair fresh water. Then put them into the honey and boil them in a pot with [a] moderate fire the space of quarter of an hour or less. Take them from the fire, skimming them well.

TO CONFIT PEACHES AFTER THE
SPANISH FASHION

Take great and fair peaches and peel them clean. Cut them in pieces, and so lay them upon a table abroad in the sun the space of two days, turning them every morning and night. Put them hot into a julep* of sugar, well sodden and prepared as is aforesaid. And after you have taken them out, set them in again in the sun, turning them often, until they be well dried. This done, put them again into the julep. Then set them in the sun until they have gotten a fair bark or crust. Then you may keep them in boxes for winter.

* *A syrup.*

A GOODLY SECRET FOR TO CONDITE OR CONFIT
ORANGES, CITRONS, AND ALL OTHER FRUITS IN SYRUP

Take citrons and cut them in pieces, taking out of them the juice or substance. Then boil them in fresh water half an hour, until they be tender. When you take them out cast them in cold water. Leave them there a good while. Then set them on the fire again in other fresh water. Do but heat it a little with a small fire, for it must not seethe, but let it simper a little. Continue thus eight days together, heating them every day in hot water. Some heat the water but one day, to the end the citrons be not too tender, but change the fresh water at night to take out the bitterness of the peels. The which, being taken away, you must take sugar or honey, clarified, wherein you must the citrons put, having first dried them from the water. In winter you must keep them from the frost, and in summer you shall leave them there all night, and a day and a night, in honey. Then boil the honey or sugar by itself, without the oranges or citrons, by the space of half an hour or less, with a little fire. And being cold, set it again to the fire with the citrons, continuing so two mornings.If you will put honey in water and not sugar, you must clarify it two times and strain it through a strainer. Having thus warmed and clarified it, you shall strain and set it again to the fire, with citrons only, making them to boil with a soft fire the space of a quarter of an hour. Then take it from the fire and let it rest at every time you do it, a day and a night. At the next morning you shall boil it again together the space of half an hour, and do for two mornings, to the end that the honey or sugar may be well incorporated with the citrons. All the cunning consisteth in the boiling of this syrup together with the citrons, and also the syrup by itself. Herein heed must be taken that it take not the smoke, so that it savour not of the fire. In this manner may be dressed the peaches, or lemons, oranges, apples, green walnuts, and other like, being boiled more or less, according to the nature of the fruits.

TO MAKE CONSERVE OF ROSES AND OF
ANY OTHER FLOWERS

Take your roses before they be fully sprung out, and chop off the white of them. Let the roses be dried one day or two before they be stamped. To one ounce of these flowers take one ounce and a half of fine beaten sugar. Let your roses be beaten as [hard as] you can, and after beat your roses and sugar together again. Then put the conserve into a fair glass. Likewise make all conserve of flowers.

TO MAKE CONSERVE OF CHERRIES
AND OTHER FRUITS

Take half a pound of cherries, and boil them dry in their own liquor. Then strain them through a hearne rafe,* and when you have strained them, put in two pounds of fine beaten sugar, and boil them together a pretty while. Then put your conserve in a pot.
* *Hair sieve.*

TO PRESERVE GOOSEBERRIES

Take to every pound of gooseberries one pound of sugar. Then take some of the gooseberries and strain them. Then take the syrup, and to every pound of gooseberries take half a pound of syrup. Then set the sugar and the syrup over the fire, and put in the gooseberries, and boil them four several times, and skim them clean.

TO PRESERVE ALL KINDS OF FRUITS, THAT THEY SHALL NOT BREAK IN THE PRESERVING OF THEM

Take a platter that is plain in the bottom, and lay sugar in the bottom, then cherries or any other fruit. And so between every row you lay, throw sugar. And set it upon a pots head, and cover it with a dish, and so let it boil.

VEGETABLES

SALADS

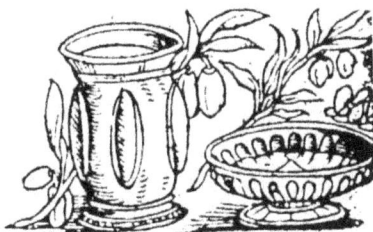

TO MAKE A SALLET OF LEMONS

Cut out slices of the peel of the lemons, longways, a quarter of an inch one piece from another. Then slice the lemon very thin and lay him an a dish cross[ways]. The peels about the lemons. Scrape a good deal of sugar on them and so serve them.

TO MAKE A DISH OF ARTICHOKES

Take your artichokes and pare away all the top, even to the meat,and boil them in sweet broth till they be somewhat tender. Then take them out and put them into a dish and seethe them with pepper, cinnamon and ginger. Then put in your dish that you mean to bake them in, and put in marrow good store, and so let them bake. And when they be baked put in a little vinegar and butter. Stick three or four leaves of the artichokes in the dish when you serve them up, and scrape sugar on the dish.

TO MAKE A SALLET OF ALL KIND OF HERBS

Take your herbs and pick them very fine into fair water, and pick your flowers by themselves. Wash them all clean, and swing them in a strainer, and when you put them into a dish, mingle them with cucumbers or lemons, pared and sliced. And scrape sugar, and put in vinegar and oil, and throw the flowers on top of the salad, and garnish the dish about of every sort of the aforesaid things, and hard eggs, boiled, and laid about the dish and upon the salad.

TO MAKE PEASCODS IN LENT

Take figs, raisins, and a few dates, and beat them very fine. And season it with cloves, mace, cinnamon and ginger.

For your paste seethe fair water and oil in a dish upon coals, and put therein saffron and salt and a little flour. Fashion them like peascods, and when you will serve them, fry them in oil in a frying pan. Let your oil be very hot, and the fire soft for burning of them. When you make them for flesh days take a fillet of veal and mince it fine, and put in the yolks of two or three raw eggs to it. Season it with pepper, salt, cloves, mace, honey, sugar,cinnamon, ginger, small raisins or great, minced. And for your paste , butter, the yolk of an egg. Season them, and fry them in butter as you did the other in oil.

TO MAKE FRIED TOAST OF SPINACH

Take spinach and seethe it in water and salt. When it is tender, wring out the water between two trenchers. Then chop it small and set it on a chafing dish of coals. Put thereto butter, small raisins, cinnamon, ginger, sugar, a little of the juice of an orange, and two yolks of raw eggs. Let it boil till it be somewhat thick. Then toast your toast, soak them in a little butter and sugar and spread thin your spinach upon them. Set them on a dish before the fire a little while. So serve them with a little sugar upon them.

A SOP OF ONIONS

Take and slice your onions and put them in a frying pan with a dish or two of sweet butter, and fry them together. Then take a little fair water and put into it salt and pepper, and so fry them together a little more. Then boil them in a little earthen pot, putting to it a little water and sweet butter. And you may use spinach in like manner.

SALLETS FOR FISH DAYS

First a salad of green fine herbs, putting periwinkles among them, with oil and vinegar.

ANOTHER

Olives and capers in one dish with vinegar and oil.

ANOTHER

White endive in a dish with periwinkles upon it, and oil and vinegar.

ANOTHER

Carrot roots being minced, and then made in the dish, after the proportion of a flowerdeluce.* Then pick shrimps and lay upon it with oil and vinegar.
* *Flower de luce, Fleur de lys. Iris pseudocorus.*

ANOTHER

Onions in flakes laid round about the dish, with minced carrots laid in the middle of the dish: wih boiled hips in five parts, like an oak leaf: made and garnished with tawney*, long cut, with oil and vinegar.
* *Tunny.*

ANOTHER

Alexander buds cut long ways garnished with whelks.

ANOTHER

Skirret* roots cut long ways, with tawney, long cut, vinegar and oil.
* *A kind of parsnip, cooked the same way as salsify. Sium sisarum.*

ANOTHER

Salmon cut long ways, with slices of onions laid upon it, and upon that to cast violets, oil and vinegar.

ANOTHER

Take pickled herrings cut long ways, and lay then in roundels, with onions and parsley, chopped. Other herrings, the bones being taken out, to be chopped together, and laid in the roundels, with a long piece laid betwixt the roundels like the proportion of a snake: garnished with tawney, long cut, with vinegar and oil.

ANOTHER

Take pickled herrings and cut them long ways, and so lay them in a dish and serve them with oil and vinegar.

TO MAKE A GALANTINE* FOR FLESH OR FISH

Take brown bread and burn it black in the toasting of it. Then take them and lay them in a little wine and vinegar, and when they have soaked a while, then strain them, seasoning it with cinnamon, ginger, pepper, and salt. Then set it on a chafing dish with coals, and let it boil till it be thick, and then serve it in saucers.
* *A strong sauce.*

A SAUCE FOR A CONEY

Cut onions in roundels and fry them in butter. Then put to them wine vinegar, salt, ginger, camomile, and pepper, and a little sugar, and let it boil till it be good and fast. Then serve it upon the coney.

BANQUETING FOOD

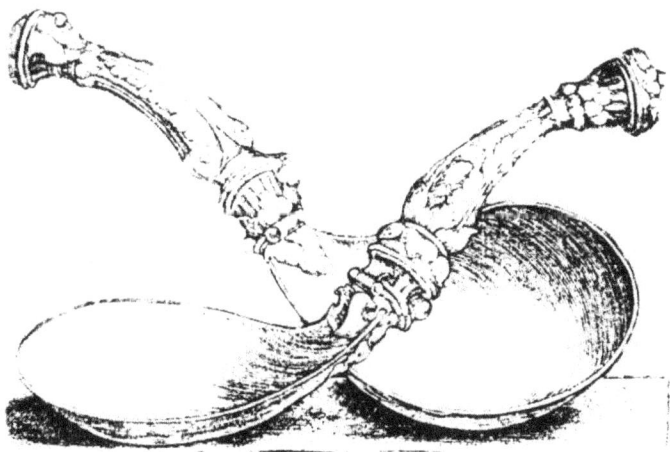

THE NAMES OF ALL THINGS NECESSARY
FOR A BANQUET

Sugar: Cinnamon: Liquorice: Pepper: Nutmegs: Saffron: Saunders:* all kinds of Comfits: Aniseeds: Coriander: Oranges: Pomegranate Seeds: [Illegible] Damask water: Lemons: Prunes: Rose water: Dates: Currants: Raisins: Cherries, conserved: Barberries, conserved: Rye flour: Ginger: Sweet oranges: Pepper, white and brown: Cloves: Mace: Wafers: For your marchpanes,** seasoned and unseasoned spinach.

* *Colouring, comes from Sanders Blue, a corruption of the French cendres bleu, azurite.*

** *Marzipan.*

TO MAKE A PASTE OF SUGAR, WHERE
OF A MAN MAY MAKE ALL MANNER OF
FRUITS, AND OTHER FINE THINGS
WITH THEIR FORM, AS PLATES,
DISHES, CUPS, AND SUCHLIKE THINGS,
WHEREWITH YOU MAY FURNISH A TABLE

Take gum and dragant,* as much as you will, and steep it in rose water till it be mollified. For four ounces of sugar take of it the bigness of a bean; the juice of lemons, a walnut shell full, and a little of the white of an egg. But you must first take the gum, and beat it so much with a pestle in a brazen mortar till it become like water. Then put to it the juice with the white of an egg, incorporating all these well together. This done, take four ounces of fine white sugar, well beaten to powder, and cast it into the said mortar by little and little, until they be turned into the form of paste. Then take it out of the mortar and bray it upon the powder of sugar, as if it were meal or flour, until it be like soft paste; to the end you may turn it and fashion it which way you will.
* *Gum tragacanth, from Middle East shrubs of genus Astragalus.*

When you have brought your paste to this form, spread it abroad upon great or small leaves, as you shall think it good. So shall you form or make what things you will, as is aforesaid, with such fine knacks as may serve a table, taking heed there stand no hot thing nigh it.

At the end of the banquet they may eat all, and break the platters, dishes, glasses, cups, and all other things, for this paste is very delicate and savorous. If you will make a thing of more finess than this, make a tart of almonds stamped with sugar and rose water, of like sort that marchpanes be made of. This shall you lay between two pastes of such vessels or fruits, or some other things, as you think good.

TO FARCE A CABBAGE FOR A BANQUET DISH

Take [a] little round cabbage, cutting off the stalks. Then make a round hole in your cabbage, as much as will receive your farcing meat, take heed you break not the brims thereof with your knife, for the hole must be round and deep. Then take the kidney of a mutton or more, and chop it not small. Then boil six eggs, hard, taking the yolks of them being small chopped. And also take raw eggs and a manchet, grated fine. Then take a handful of prunes, so many great raisins, seasoning all these with salt, pepper, cloves and mace, working all these together. And so stuff your cabbage. But if you have sausage you may put it among your meat at the putting in of your stuff. But you must leave out both ends of your sausage at the mouth of the cabbage when you shall serve it out. In the boiling it must be within the cabbage, and the cabbage must be stopped close with his cover in the time of his boiling, and bound fast round about for breaking. The cabbage must be sod in a deep pot with fresh beef broth or mutton broth, and no more than will lie unto the top of the cabbage. When it is enough, take away the thread, and so set it in a platter, opening the head and laying out the sausage ends. And so serve it forth.

TO MAKE A SPREAD EAGLE OF A PULLET

Take a good pullet and cut his throat hard by the head, and make it but a little hole. Then scald him clean, and take out of the small hole his crop. So done, take a quill and blow into the same hole, for to make the skin to rise from the flesh. Then break the wing bones, and the bones hard by the knee. Then cut the neck hard by the body within the skin: then cut off the rump within the skin, leaving the bones at the legs, and also the head on. So drawing the whole body out within the skin of the hole. The bones to be laid beneath towards the claws, and the feet being left also on. You must cut off his bill. When you have taken out all these bones and brought it to the purpose, then take the flesh of the same pullet and parboil it a little, and mince it fine with sheep's suet, grated bread and three yolks of hard eggs. Then bind it with four raw eggs, and a few barberries, working these together. Season it with cloves, mace, ginger, pepper and salt, and saffron. Then stuff your pullet's skin with it, putting it in at the hole at the head. When you have stuffed him, take him and lay him flat in a platter, and make it after the proportion of an eagle in every part, having his head to be cleft asunder and laid in two parts like an eagle's head. Thus done, then must you put him into the oven, leaving in the platter a dish of butter underneath him, [and] another upon him because of burning. And when it is enough, then set it forth, casting upon him in the service, blanch powder, made of cinnamon, ginger and sugar.

TO BOIL A PIKE WITH ORANGES
A BANQUET DISH

Take your pike, split him, and seethe him alone with water, butter, and salt. Then take an earthen pot and put into it a pint of water and another of wine, with two oranges or two lemons if you have them. If not, then take four or five oranges, the rinds being cut away and sliced, and so put to the liquor, with six dates cut long ways. Season your broth with ginger, pepper and salt, and two dishes of sweet butter, boiling these together. And when you will serve him, lay your pike upon sops, casting your broth upon it. You must remember that you cut off your pike's head hard by the body, and then his body to be splitted, cutting every side in two or three parts, and when he is enough, setting the body of the fish in order. Then take his head and set it at the foremost part of the dish, standing upright with an orange in his mouth.

TO BRAY GOLD

Take gold leaves, four drops of honey, mix it well together, and put it into a glass. And when you will occupy it, steep and temper it in gum water. And it will be good.

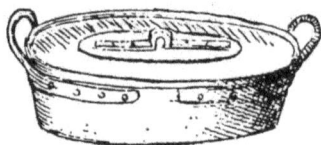

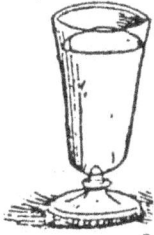

THREE

DRINKS

TO MAKE A CAUDLE

Take a pint of malmsey and five or six eggs, and seethe them, strained, together. So sodden, stir it till it be thick. Lay it in a dish as you do please and so serve it.

TO MAKE A CAUDLE OF OATMEAL

Take two handfuls or more of great oatmeal and beat it in a stone mortar, well. Then put it into a quart of ale, and set it on the fire and stir it. Season it with cloves, mace, and sugar, beaten, and let it boil till it be enough. Then serve it forth upon sops.

TO MAKE HYPOCRACE*

Take a gallon of white wine, sugar two pounds, of cinnamon, ginger, long pepper, mace not bruised, grains** galingall.*** yd.od. and cloves, not bruised. You must bruise every kind of spice a little and put them in an earthen pot all day. And then cast them through your bags two times or more as you see cause. And so drink it.
* *A spiced drink of red wine said to have been invented by Hippocrates. In Dawson's version a white wine drink.*
** *These spices have y.d. after them meaning either y-diced, or y-drawn — that is, drawn through a strainer.*
*** *Rhyzome of the ginger family.*

123

HUSBANDRY

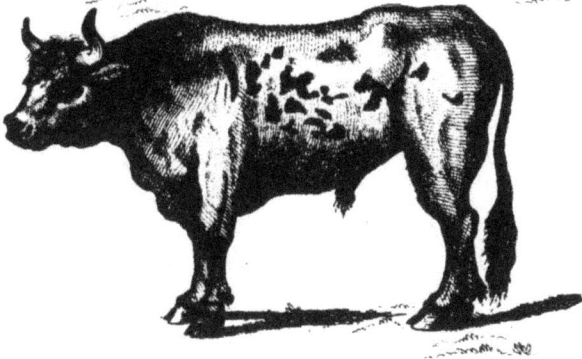

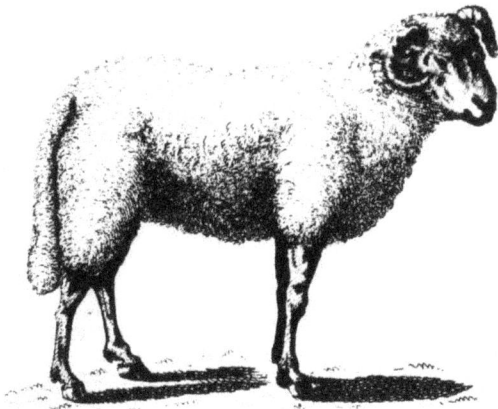

CERTAIN APPROVED POINTS OF HUSBANDRY, VERY NECESSARY FOR ALL HUSBANDMEN TO KNOW

FIRST OF OXEN

Tokens whereby an ox is known to be good and toward for the work are these:

Ready and quick at the voice, he moveth quickly, he is short and large, great ears, the horns lively and of mean bigness and black, the head short, the breast large, a great paunch, the tail long, touching the ground with a tuft at the end, the hair curled, the back straight, the reins* large, the leg strong and sinuous, the hoof short and large. The best colour is black and red, and next unto that the bay and the pied. The white is the worst. The grey and the fallow or yellow is of less value.

The charge of one that keepeth them is chiefly to use them gently, to serve them with meat** and good litter, to rub or comb them at night, to strike*** them over in the morning, washing sometimes their tails in warm water. Also to keep their stable clean, that the poultry and hogs come not in, for the feathers may kill the Oxen, and the dung of sick hogs breedeth the murren.

Item. He must know discreetly when oxen have laboured enough, and when but little, according to that they are to be fed.

Item. That he work them not in a time too cold or too wet.

Item. That he suffer them not to drink presently after great labour, and that he tie them not up forthwith until they be a little refreshed abroad.

* *Kidneys*
** *Food.*
*** *Rub.*

The ox desireth clear or running water like as the Horse desireth the puddle or troughed water.

Item. That at their coming home he always over look them, whether there be any thorns in their feet, or if the yolk hath galled them.

In France they geld all their bull calves about the age of two years, and that at the fall of the leaf.

The day they are to be cut, they must not drink, and must eat but little. They suddenly clip the sinews of the stones with a pair of tongs. And so cut out the stones in such sort as they leave behind the end that is tied unto the sinews for so the calf or bullock shall not bleed overmuch, nor shall loose all his virility and courage.

At the age of ten months the bullock changeth his foreteeth, and at six months after they scale the next teeth. And at the end of three years he changeth all his teeth.

Note. When an ox is at best, his teeth are equal, white and long, and when he is old, the teeth be unequal and black.

If an ox have the lask,* which often times is with blood and maketh him very weak, they keep him from drink four or five days. They give him walnuts and hard cheese tempered in thick wine. For the uttermost remedy they let him bleed in the middle of the forehead.

To make him loose bellied they give him two ounces of aloes, made in powder with warm water.

An ox pisseth blood of being too much chafed, or of eating ill herbs or flowers. They keep him from drink and drench him with treacle in two pints of wine or ale, putting thereto saffron.

For the cough they seethe hyssop in his drink.

For the biting of an adder or venomous dog, they anoint the place with oil of scorpion.

If he be lame of cold in his feet, they wash him with old brine, warmed.

* *Diarrhoea.*

If he be lame of the abundance of blood fallen down into the pastornes* and hoof, they dissolve it by rubbing and lancing.

Item. The better to keep their oxen in health, whether they are to be laboured or to be fatted, they wash his mouth eight days with brine, and there is taken away much fleame,** which taketh from an ox his taste and stomach.

If the fleame have made him have the murre*** which is known by the watering of the eye, they wash his mouth with thyme and white wine or rub it with water and salt.

* *Pasterns*
** *Phlegm.*
*** *An infectious disease of cattle.*

OF HORSES

Tokens of a good colt:

The head little and lean, the ear straight, the eyes great, the nostrils wide, the neck little towards the head, the back short and large, close bellied, the cultions or stones equal and small, the tail long, tufted with hair thick and curled, the legs equal, high and straight, the hoof black, hard and high. He should be quick and pleasant.

The age of the horses is known partly by the hoof, and principally by the teeth. When the horse is two years and a half the middle teeth above and beneath do fall.

When he is four years old the dog teeth fall and others come in their places. Before he be six years old the great teeth above do fall. And the sixth year the first that fell do come again. The seventh year all is full and they be all shut.

OF SHEEP

Certain days before the rams be put to the ewes, they drench them with salt water; thereby the ewes will take the better, and the rams (they say) wax more full of appetite.

To have many male lambs they choose a dry time, the wind at north. Letting the ewes go in pasture that lieth open against the northen wind. And then put in the rams.

To have many female lambs they contrarywise observe the south wind.

When a ewe is with lamb, if she have a black tongue, they say the lamb will be black. And if the tongue be white, the lamb, likewise, will be white.

Tokens of a good Sheep: A great body, the neck long, the wool deep, soft, and fine. The belly great, and covered with wool, the teats great, great eyes, long legs and long tail.

Tokens of a good Ram: The body high and long, a great belly covered with wool, a fleece thick. The forehead broad, eyes black with much well about them, great ears covered with wool, great stones, well horned,but the more writhed the better. The tongue and pallet of the mouth all white, to the end that the lambs may be all white.

APPROVED POINTS OF HOGS

The hog of himself though filthy, yet, they say, prospereth the best if he lodge ina clean stye. And every month his stye should be cast over with fresh gravel or sand, to make his lying fresh and to dry up the piss and filth.

They geld their pigs when they are a year old or six months at the least, for they wax much greater if they be gelded at the said age.

They choose them boars that have the head short and large, the breast large, colour black or white, the feet short, the legs great, and those that have strongest hair on top of their back.

Those are to kept for sows which be longest, with hanging bellies, great teats, deep ribbed, a little head and short legs.

Hogs be sick when they rub much their ears or refrain their meat, but if none of these signs appear, they pluck off one of his hairs on the back. If he be clean and white at the root, he is well. If he be bloody or foul he is sick.

They will have their hogs either all white or all black, and in any wise not speckled or of two colours.

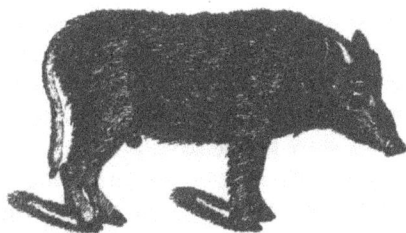

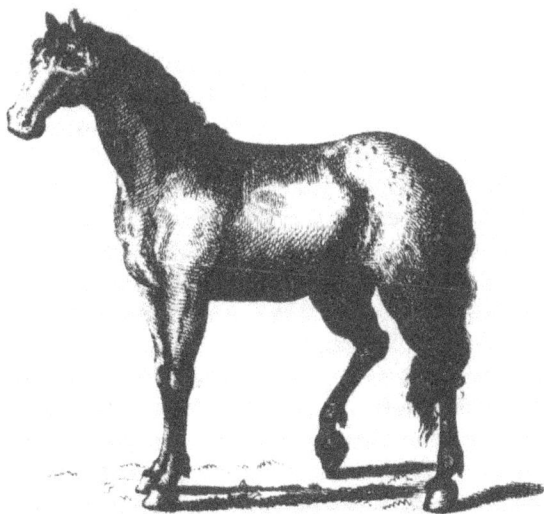

They refrain from dunging their land while the moon increaseth, for that they note more abundance of weeds to come up thereby.

Touching the sowing of beans they observe this: At the fall of the leaf in strong land they sow the great beans. At Spring time in weak and round ground they sow the common small beans, and both sorts at the full of the moon, that they may be better codded. They use to cut them at the new of the moon before day. Their flax, as soon as they have gathered it, they set it under a house or hovel and suffer it not to take rain or dew as we do.

To make cheese yellow they put in a little saffron.

To keep apples they lay them on straw strewed. The eye of the apple downwards and not the stem. When they would have any great store, well and long kept from perishing, they gather and choose the soundest, heaviest, and fairest, being not over riped, they provide a hogshead, fat, or great whitch.* They bring the apples where it shall stand. Then they lay a laine** of straw and upon the same a line of apples, and then straw again and apples likewise, until the vessel be full to the brim, shutting it close with the head or cover that no air come in.

To cure the malady of trees that bear worm eaten fruit, which cometh of much wet or a moist season. At that time they pierce the trees through with an augur as near the root as they may, to the end that the humour whereof the worms do breed may distil out of the tree. If trees through oldness or otherwise leave bearing of fruit, usually they use not to lop them, but only cut away the head boughs. They uncover the roots after All Saints tide, and cleave the greatest of the roots, putting into the clefts shivers of flints or hard stones, letting them there remain. To the end that the humour of the earth may enter and ascend into the tree after the end of the winter. They cover again the roots with very good earth. If they have any dead carrions they bury them about the roots of such trees.

* *Box or coffin*
* **Layer.*

132

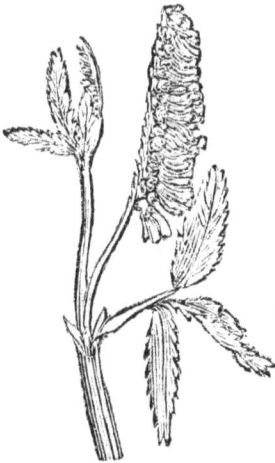

Melilot.

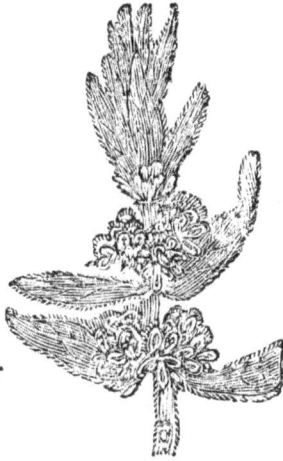

Mother-wort.

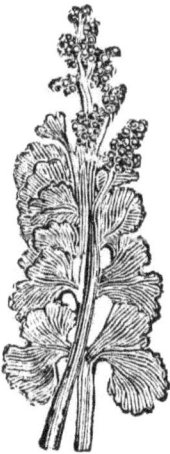

Moon-wort.

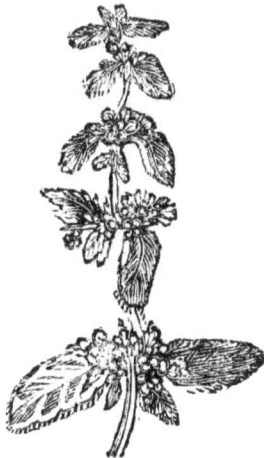

Pennyroyal.

REMEDIES

Advice from a qualified herablist should be asked before using these recipes.

TO MAKE STRONG BROTH FOR A SICK MAN

Take a pound of almonds and blanch them, and beat them in a very fine mortar. Then take the brains of a capon and beat with it. Put in to it a little cream and make it to draw through a strainer. Then set it on the fire in a dish, and season it with rose water and sugar, and stir it.

TO MAKE A TART THAT IS COURAGE TO A MAN OR WOMAN

Take two quinces and two or three bur* roots, and a potato, and pare your potato and scrape your roots, and put them into a quart of wine. Let them boil till they be tender. And put in an ounce of dates. When they be boiled tender draw them through a strainer, wine and all, and then put in the yolks of eight eggs, and the brains of three or four cock sparrows, and strain them into the other, and a little rose water. Seethe them all with sugar, cinnamon and ginger, cloves and mace. Put in a little sweet butter, and set it upon a chafing dish of coals between two platters. And so let it boil till it be something big.
* Burdock.

TO MAKE A CAUDLE TO COMFORT THE STOMACH, GOOD FOR AN OLD MAN

Take a pint of good muscadine, and as much of good stale ale, mingle them together. Then take the yolks of twelve or thirteen eggs, new laid. Beat well the eggs, first by themselves, [then] with the wine and ale, and so boil it together. And put thereto a quartern of sugar, and a few whole mace, and so stir it well, till it seethe a good while.

135

When it is well sod, put therein a few slices of bread if you will. And so let it soak a while, and it will be right good and wholesome.

TO MAKE POTTAGE TO LOOSE THE BODY

Take a chicken and seethe it in running water, then take two handfuls of violet leaves, and a good pretty sort of raisins of the sun, pick out the stones, and seethe them with the chickens. When it is well sodden, season it with a little salt and strain it and serve it.

TO MAKE ANOTHER VERY GOOD POTTAGE TO BE USED IN THE MORNING

Take a chicken and seethe it in fair water and put to it violet leaves, a handful or two, or else some other good herbs that you like instead of them. So let them seethe together till the Chicken be ready to fall to pieces. Then strain it, and cut thin pieces of bread, and seethe in it till the bread be very tender, and then season it with salt. And on the fifth day seethe the herbs as before in fair running water, and strain it, and seethe bread as before in it. Season it with salt and put in a piece of butter.

TO MAKE BROTH FOR ONE THAT IS WEAK

Take a leg of veal and set it over the fire in a gallon of water, skimming it clean. When you have done so, put in three quarters of a pound of small raisins, half a pound of prunes, a good handful of borage, as much langdebeef,* as much mints, and a like quantity of harts-tongue. Let all seethe together till all the strength of the flesh be sodden out. Then strain it so clean as you can. If you think the

patient be in any heat, put in violet leaves and savory as you
do with the other herbs.
* *Borage.*

TO MAKE A SYRUP OF QUINCES TO
COMFORT THE STOMACH

Take a great pint of the juice of quinces, a pound of sugar,
and a good half pint of vinegar, of ginger the weight of five
groats, of cinnamon the weight of six groats, of pepper the
weight of three groats and two pence.

A POWDER PEERLESS FOR WOUNDS

Take orpiment* and verdigris, of each an ounce, of vitriol
burned till it be red, two ounces, bray* each of them by it self
in a brazen mortar, as small as flour. Then mingle them
altogether that they appear all as one. Keep it in bags of
leather, well bound, for it will last seven years with one
virtue. It is called powder peerless, it hath no peer for
working in surgery, for to put this powder in a wound,
whereas is dead flesh, and lay scraped** lint about it,(and a
plaster of duiflosius next underneath written, and it etc. The
rest wanteth).
* *Arsenic trisulphate.*
** *Beat*

A MEDICINE FOR THE MEGRIME,
IMPOSTUME OF THE REWME, OR OTHER
DISEASES IN THE HEAD

Take pellitory of Spain,* the weight of a groat, half so
much spegall,** and beat these in powder, take the tops of
hyssop, of rosemary with the flowers, three or four leaves of
* *Anacyclus pyrethrum, an irritant and salivant.*
** *Spignall or spikenard.*

sage in the bole, of these herbs one small handful. Boil all these herbs with the spices in half a pint of white wine, and half a pint of vinegar of roses, until one half of the liquor be consumed. Then strain forth the herbs and set the liquor to cool. And being cold put thereunto three spoonfuls of good mustard, and so much honey as will take away the tartness of the medicine. When the patient feeleth any pain in his head take a spoonful thereofand put it into his mouth and hold it a pretty while gargling. Then spitteth it forth into a vessel. And so use: take ten spoonfuls at one time in the morning, fasting, using this three days together, when they feel themselves troubled with the rewme. At the fall and spring of the leaf is best taking thereof. And by the grace of God they shall find ease.

You must keep this same medicine very close in a glass. Whole goodness will last ten days. When you take it warm it as milk from the cow.

A COPY OF DOCTOR STEVENS WATER

Take a gallon of Gascoigne wine, then take ginger, galingale, camomile,cinnamon, grain, cloves, mace, aniseeds,fennel seeds, carraway seeds, of every one one dram, that is two pence halfpenny weight. Then take sugar, minced, red roses, thyme, pellitory of the wall,* wild marjoram, penny royal, pennymountain, wild thyme, lavender, avens,** of every of them one handful. Then beat the spice small, and bruise the herbs, and put all to the wine, and let it stand twelve hours, stirring it at divers times. Then still it in a limbecke.*** Keep the first pint of water by it self, so it is best. Then will come a second water, which is not so good as the first. The virtue of this water is this; it comforteth the spirits and preserveth greatly the youth of man, and helpeth inward diseases coming of cold, against the shaking of the palsey, it cureth the contraction of sinews, and helpeth the conception of women, it killeth the worms in the belly, it helpeth the toothache, it helpeth the cold gout, it comforteth the stomach, it cureth the cold dropsy, it helpeth the stone in the bladder, and the reins**** of the back, it cureth the canker, it helpeth, shortly, a stinking breath. And who so useth this water now and then and not too often, it preserveth him a good liking, and shall make him seem young very long.

* *Parietaria officinalis.*
** *Colewort or herb bonet.*
*** *Alembic still. A close vessel for distilling.*
**** *Kidneys.*

A MEDICINE FOR ALL MANNER OF SORES

Take unwrought ware,* turpentine, oil olive, sheep's tallow or deer's suet, a quantity of every of them. Then take a quantity of juice of bugle,** the juice of smallage,*** a quantity of rosin, and boil them all together over a soft fire. Stirring them always till they be well mingled, and that the greeness of the juice be come. Then strain it through a fair cloth into a clean vessel. And this shall heal wounds or sores whatsoever they be.

* *Seaweed.*
** *Bugloss.*
*** *Parsley or celery.*

ANOTHER FOR ALL SORES

Take a quarter of a pound of pitch, as much of ware, as much of rosin, as much of capons grease or other soft grease, and put them in a pan and seethe them all together till they be melted. Then strain them through a fair cloth, and make a plaster to lay them on the place grieved.

TO DEFEND HUMOURS

Take beans, the rind or upper skin being pulled off, and bruise them and mingle them with the white of an egg. Make it stick to the temples; it keepeth back humours flowing to the eyes.

TO MAKE ROSEMARY WATER

Take the rosemary and the flowers in the middle of May, before sunrise, and strip the leaves and flowers from the stalk. Take four or five alicompane * roots, and a handful or two of sage. Then beat the rosemary, the sage, and roots together till they be very small. Take three ounces of cloves, three ounces of mace, three ounces of ouibles,** half a pound of aniseeds, and beat these spices, every one by itself. Then take all the herbs and spices and put therein four or five gallons of good white wine. Then put in all these herbs and spices and wine, into an earthen pot, and put the same pot in the ground the space of thirteen days. Then take it up· and still in a still with a very soft fire.

* *Elecompane. Enulae campanae helenij.*
** *A type of wafer, from the French oublie.*

AN EXCELLENT DRINK FOR THE TISSICK*, WELL APPROVED

Take a handful of fennel roots, as much parsley roots, as many alexander roots, and half a handful of borage roots. Put out the pith of all the said roots. Then take half a handful of pennyroyal, as much of violet leaves, and as much of cinquefoil, as much of succory,** endive, hollyhocks leaves, mallow leaves, and red garden mints. Of all these the like quantity as of these next before: Half a handful of liquorice

* *Consumption.*
** *Chicory.*

sticks, scraped, bruised and beaten to fine powder, [and] a gallon of fair running water. Boil therein all these simples, and boil these seeds with them, that is, three spoonfuls of aniseeds, as much fennel seed, the like of coriander seeds, and cumin seed, a good handful of dandelion roots, and so boil altogether from a gallon to a pottell.* Let the patient drink thereof first and last, and it will help him in a short space. Probatum est.

* *Two quarts.*

TO MAKE WATER IMPERIAL FOR ALL WOUNDS AND CANKERS

Take a handful of red sage leaves, a handful of celandine, as much of woodbine leaves. Take a gallon of conduit water and put the herbs in it, and let them boil in a pottle. Then strain the herbs through a strainer, and take the liquor and set it over the fire again. Take a pint of English honey, a good handful of roche allam,* as much of white copperas,** lime beaten, a pennyworth of grains bruised, and let them boil altogether three or four warwmes.*** Then let the scum be taken off with a feather, and when it is cold put it in an earthen pot or bottle, so as it may be kept close. For a green wound take of the thinnest, and for an old wound of the thickest. Cover the sore rather with veal or mutton. Skim them with dock leaves when you have dressed them with this water.

* *Rock alum.*
** *Photosulphate of copper, iron or zinc.*
*** *Periods of boiling.*

TO MAKE WATER IMPERIAL ANOTHER WAY

Take a handful of dragon*, of scabious, of endive, a handful of pimpernell a handful of wormwood, of rue, of
* *Toadflax.*

tansy, of feverfew, of daisy leaves, of cowslips, of maidenhair, of cinquefoil, of dandelion, of thyme, of balm, of each of these herbs a handful. Of treacle, a pound, of bolearmoniacke** four ounces, and when you have all these herbs together you must take and shred them a little, not too small. Then take the treacle and the bolearmoniacke and mingle them and the herbs together. Then put them in a stillatory and still them: & fiet.

** *Astringent earth from Armenia, used as styptic or antidote.*

TO MAKE CINNAMON WATER

Take Rhenish wine, a quart, or Spanish wine, a pint: rose water a pint and a half: cinnamon , bruised, a pound and a half. Let these stand infused the space of four and twenty hours. Then distil it, and being close stopped and luted,* then with a soft fire distil the same softly in a limbeck of glass and receive the first water by itself. Also if you be so disposed to make the same water weaker, take three pints of rose water, a pint and a half of Rhenish wine and so distil the same, and you shall have to the quality of stuff, the quantity of the water, which is three pints. But the first is best, and so reserve it to your use both morning and evening.

* *Clay to make the stopping very airtight.*

TO MAKE CINNAMON WATER ANOTHER WAY

Take three quarters of muscadine, a pound of cinnamon and half a pint of good rose water, and so let them lie infused the space of four and twenty hours. Distil it as aforesaid, and you shall receive to the quantity as to the quality. But the first pint is the best and choisest of all. The other is as manifest by practise.

TO MAKE AQUA COMPOSITA FOR A SURFEIT

Take rosemary, fennel, hyssop, thyme, sage, horehound, of each of these a handful, pennyroyal, red mints, marjoram, of each six crops, a root of enula campana, of liquoris,anniseeds bruised, of each two ounces. Put all these to three gallons of mighty strong ale, and put it into a brass pot over an easy fire, and set the limbeck upon it. Stop it close with dough or paste that no air do go out. And so keep it stilling with a soft fire, and so preserve to your use as need require it.

TO MAKE WATER OF LIFE

Take balm leaves and stalks, burnet leaves and flowers, a handful of rosemary, turmentil* leaves and roots, rosasolis** a handful: red roses, a handful: carnations, a handful: hyssop, a handful: a handful of thyme: red strings that grow upon savory, a handful: red fennel leaves and roots , a handful: red mints, a handful: red fennel, a handful. Put all these herbs into a pot of earth glazed, and put thereto as much white wine as will cover the herbs. And let them soak therein eight or nine days. Then take an ounce of cinnamon, as much of ginger, as much of nutmegs, cloves and saffron, a little quantity: of anniseeds, a pound: great raisins, a pound, sugar, a pound, half a pound of dates, the hinder part of an old coney: a good fleshy running capon: the flesh and sinews of a leg of mutton: four young pigeons: a dozen of larks: the yolks of twelve eggs: a loaf of white bread cut in sippets: muscatell or bastard, three gallons, or as much quantity as sufficeth to distil all these together at once in a limbeck and thereto put of methridatum*** two or three ounces, or else with as much perfect treacle, and distil it with a moderate

* *Potentilla tormentilla.*

** *Sundew, Drosera rotundifolia.*

*** *Mustard, Lepidium campestre, or Bastard Mithridate mustard, candytuft.*

fire. Keep the first water by itself. And the second water also. And when there cometh no more water with strings, take away the limbeck and put into the pot more wine upon the same stuff, and still it again. And you shall have another good water, and shall so remain good. In the first ingredience of this water you must keep a double glass merely, for it is restorative of all principal members, and defendeth against all pestilential diseases, as against the palsy, dropsy, spleen, yellow or black jaundice, for worms in the belly, and for all agues be they hot or cold, and all manners of swellings and pestilential sorrows in man. As melancholy, and phlegmatic, and it strenghteneth and comforteth all the spirits and strings of the brain, as the heart, the milte,**** the liver and the stomach, by taking thereof two or three spoonfuls at one time by itself, or with ale, wine or beer, and by putting a pretty quantity of sugar therein. Also it helpeth digestion, and doth break wind, and stoppeth laske, and bindeth not. It mightily helpeth and saveth man or woman of the pain of the heart burning, and for to quicken the memory of man. Take of this water three spoonfuls a day, in the morning, and another after he goeth to dinner, and the third last at night.
**** *Spleen.*

TO MAKE GOOD PLASTER FOR THE STRANGURIE*

Take hollyhocks, violets and mercury, the leaves of these herbs or the seeds of them. Also the rind of the elder tree, and also leyd wort, of each of these a handful. Beat them small and seethe them in water till half be consumed. Then do thereto a little olive oil, and all hot make thereof a plaster and lay it to the sore and reins. Also in summer thou must make him a drink in this manner: take saxifrage, and the leaves of elder, fine leaved grass, and seethe them in a pottle of stale ale, till the half be wasted. Then strain it and keep it clean, and let the sick drink thereof first and last. If you lack these herbs because of winter, then take the roots of fine
* *Disease of the urinary organs.*

leaved grass and dry them, and make thereof a powder of them. Then take oyster shells and burn them, and mingle them together and so let the sick use thereof in his pottage and drink, and it shall help him.

TO MAKE A POWDER FOR THE STONE AND STRANGUILLIAN

Take black bramble berries while they be red, the inner pitch of the ash keys, the stones of the eglantine berries cloven, rubbed from the hazelnut keys, the roots of philopendula,* of all these a like quantity: (?)** acorn kernels, the stones of sloes, of each a like quantity. Dry all these on platters in an oven till they be well beaten to powder. Then take gromel** seed, saxifrage seed, alexander seed, coriander seed, parsley seed, cumin seed, fennel seed, aniseed, of each of these a like quantity as much as is before written, and dried in like sort. Then beat all these to fine powder, and take liquorice of the best that you can get, fair scraped, as much in quantity as of all the other, and beat it fine, and mingle it with the same powder, and so keep it close that no wind come at it; using it first and last with posset drink made with white wine or ale. When you eat your pottage or other broth, put some in it if you be sore pained. And if you have any stone it will come away by slivers, and if it do so, when you think that your water begining to clear again, take this drink that followeth and it will clean your bladder, and it will leave no corruption therein.

* *Filipendula, or drop wort.*
** *There is a word missing from the text here.*
*** *Lithospermum.*

THE DRINK

Take rosemary with thyme, and seethe them in running water with as much sugar as will make it sweet from a quart to a pint. Use the quantity of your herbs according to your discretion, so that it may savour well of the herbs. And so use it nine mornings, six or seven spoonfuls at a time.

FOR THE SHINGLES, A REMEDY

Take doves dirt that is moist, and of barley meal heaped, half a pound, and stamp them well together. Do thereto half a pint of vinegar, and meddle them together. And so lay it to the sore cold. Lay wall leaves thereupon, and so let it lie three days unremoved. On the third day if need require, lay thereto a new plaster of the same, and at the most he shall be whole within three plasters.

FOR ALL MANNER OF SINEWS THAT ARE SHORTENED

Take the head of a black sheep, cammomile, sorrel leaves, sage, of each [a] handful and bray these herbs in a mortar. Then boil them altogether in water, till they be well sodden, and let them stand till they be cold. Then draw it through a strainer and so use it.

A SOVEREIGN OINTMENT FOR SHRUNKEN
SINEWS AND ACHES

Take eight swallows ready to fly out of the nest. Drive away the breeders when you take them out, and let them not touch the earth. Stamp them until the feathers cannot be perceived in a stone mortar. Put to it lavender cotton, of the strings of strawberries, the tops of mother thyme,* the tops of rosemary, of each a handful. Take all their weight of May butter, and a quart more. Then make it up in bales and put it into an earthen pot for eight days close stopped, that no air take them. Take it out, and on as soft a fire as maybe, seethe
* *Wild thyme, Thymus serpyllum.*

it so that it do but simmer. Then strain it, and so reserve it to your use.

FOR SINEWS THAT BE BROKEN IN TWO

Take worms while they be nice, and look that they depart not. Stamp them, and lay it to the sore, and it will knit the sinew that be broken in two.

FOR TO KNIT SINEWS THAT BE BROKEN

Take archangel* and cut it in small gobbets, and lay it to the sore. Take milfoil and stamp it, and lay it above it, hard bound. Let it lie so three days, and at three days end take it away and wash it with wine. Then make a new plaster of the same and at the three days end put thereto another, and do nothing else thereto. Also take pennyroyal and bray it, and put salt enough to them. Temper it with honey and make a plaster thereof, and lay it upon the sinews that be stiff and it will make them to stretch.
* *Dead nettle.*

AN OIL TO STRETCH SINEWS THAT BE SHRUNK

Take a quart of neat's foot oil and a pint of neat's gall: half a pint of rose water: as much aqua vita: then put all these together into a brass pan. Then take a handful of lavender cotton, and as much of bay leaves, a good quantity of rosemary, a good quantity of lavender spike, of strawberry leaves, the strings and all. Then take thread and bind them all in several bunches, and put them into the pan or pot. Set them over the fire upon clear coals, with the oils altogether. And so let them boil a good while. When it is boiled enough it will boil but softly. Then take it off the fire and let it stand till it be almost cold. Strain it out into a wide mouthed glass, bottle or pewter pot, and stop it close. It will not continue in no wooden thing. Where the sinews be shrunk: take of this being warmed, and annoint the place therewith, and chafe it well against the fire. Do this morning and evening, and keep the place warm, and you shall find great ease.

FOR TO STAUNCH BLOOD

Take bole armoniake and turpentine, and make a plaster, and lay it to. Take the moss of the hazel tree and cast it into the wound, and it will staunch forthwith. The longer it is gathered the better it is. Also take a good piece of Martinmas beef out of the roast, and heat it on coals, and as hot as you may suffer it, lay it thereto. Also take a piece of lean salt beef, and let the beef be of that greatness that it may fill the wound, and lay it in the fire in the hot ashes till it be hot through, and all hot stuff it in the wound and bind it fast. And it shall staunch anon the bleeding when a master vein is cut, and if the wound be large.

FOR SWELLING THAT COMETH SUDDENLY IN MAN'S LIMBS

Take harts tongue [and] chervil, and cut them small. Then take dregs of ale and wheat bran, and sheeps tallow melted, and do all in a pot. Seethe them till that they be thick. Then make a plaster and lay it to the swelling. Also take fair water and salt and stir them well together, and therein wet a cloth and lay it to the swelling.

FOR TO MAKE ONE SLENDER

Take fennel, and seethe it in water, a very good quantity, and wring out the juice thereof when it is sod. Drink it first and last and it shall assuage either him or her.

A GOOD OINTMENT FOR SCABS, AND FOR ITCHING OF THE BODY

Take four ounces of oil de baye*, and an ounce of frankincense, and two ounces of white whey, three ounces of swine's grease, and an ounce of quick silver that must be slaked with falling spittle, an ounce of great salt, as much of the one as of the other. Of all these make an ointment. If the scabs or itch be upon the whole body as well above the girdle as beneath, then when thou goest to bed wash both thy hands and thy feet with warm water, and battle them well therein by the fire. Then after dry them with a cloth of linen. Then take up with thy fingers of that ointment, and do it in the palms of thy hands, and in the soles of thy feet and rub it well together that it may drink in well. And if it does soak in well thou must put gloves on thy hands and socks on thy feet. Thus do every night when thou goest to bed. And if the scab and itch be above the girdle and not beneath, then annoint but thy hands, and if the the scab be beneath the girdle, then look that you annoint the soles of your feet. And the scab or itch be in all the body, as well above the girdle as beneath, then thou must annoint both thy hands and thy feet as thou sittest by the fire, and thou shalt be whole. This hath been proved.

* *Oil made from berries of the bay.*

FOR ALL MANNER OF SCABS

Take enela campana, red dock roots, nightshade, woodbine leaves, and then salt in a piece of alum, and put in vitriol Romana* rubrified,** when it is cold, and wash the scab therewith. Take white ointment, brimstone, quicksilver, verdisgris, and mingle them together. Therewith annoint the sore scab.

* *Sulphate of iron.*
** *Reddened.*

FOR A MAN THAT HATH DRUNKEN POISON

Take betony, and stamp it and mingle it with water. And the poison that the party hath drunk will presently come forth again.

TO RESTORE SPEECH THAT IS LOST SUDDENLY

Take pennyroyal, and temper it with aysel,* and give it to the sick to drink it. Lay also a plaster of this to his nostrils so grieved.
* *Vinegar.*

TO STILL A CAPON FOR A SICK PERSON

Take a well fleshed capon, fair scalded and dressed, and put him into an earthen pot. Put to it borage and bugloss, three handfuls of mint, one handful of harts tongue and lange de beef, [and] a handful of hyssop; and put thereto a pint of claret wine, and a pint of clean water, and twelve prunes. When you have so done, cover the pot with a dish or saucer, and upon that all to cover coarse paste, that no air come out. Then take the pot and hang in a brass pot up to the brims of your paste, and so let it boil for twelve hours at the least. And always as your water that is in your brass pot doth consume, be sure to have in readiness another pot of hot water at the fire to fill it, as long as it doth seethe for the twelve hours. When the hours be past, take it from the fire, and let it cool for one hour. Then unloose and strain the liquor from the capon into a fair pot, taking every morning, warm, four or five spoonfuls next to your heart. Which shall comfort and restore nature to you being sick, using this aforesaid capon.

THE STILLING OF A CAPON, A GREAT RESTORATIVE

Take a young capon that is well fleshed and not fat, and a knuckle of young veal that is sucking, and let not fat be upon

it, and all to hack it, bones and all. And flea* the capon, clean the skin from the flesh and quarter it in four quarters, and all to burst it, bones and all. Put the veal and it together in an earthen pot; put to it a pint of red wine, and eight spoonfuls of rose water, half a pound of small raisins and currants, four dates quartered, a handful of rosemary flowers, a handful of borage flowers, and twenty or thirty whole maces. Take and cover the pot close with a cover, and take paste and put it about the pot's mouth, that no air come forth. Set it within a brass pot full of water on the fire, and let it boil there eight hours. Then take the ladle and bruise it altogether within the pot. Put it in a fair strainer and strain it through with the ladle. Let no fat be upon the broth but that it may be blown, or else taken with a feather. And every day next your heart drink half a dozen spoonfuls thereof, with a cake of Manus Christi, and again at four of the clock in the afternoon.
* *Flay, skin.*

TO MAKE A COLLUCE

Take all the bones and legs of the aforesaid capon, hen, or pullet, and beat them fine in a stone mortar: putting to it half a pint or more of the same liquor that it was sodden in. Then strain it and put to it a little sugar. Then put it into a stone crews*, and so drink it warm first and last.
* *Cruse. A drinking vessel or bowl.*

* *

TO MAKE GOOD SOAP

First you must take half a strike* of ashen ashes and a quart of lime. Then you must mingle both these together. Then you must fill a pan full of water and seethe them well. So done, you must take four pounds of beast's tallow, and put it into the lye, and seethe them together until it be hard.
* *Cut.*

151

To make Rosemary water.

TAke the Rosemarye, and the flowers in the middest of May, before sunne arise, and strippe the leaues and the flowers from the stalke, take foure or fiue alicompane rootes, and a handfull or two of Sage, then beate the Rosemarye, the Sage and rootes together, till they be very small, and take three ounces of Cloues, iij ounces of Mace, iij ounces of Quibles, halfe a pound of Annifeedes, and beate these spices euery one by it selfe. Then take all the hearbes and the Spices, and put therein foure or fiue gallons of good white wine, then put in all these Hearbes and Spices, and Wine, into an earthen pot, and put the same pot in the ground the space of sirtæne dayes, then take it vp, and styll in a Styll with a very soft fire.

To make Bisket bread.

FIrste take halfe a Pecke of fine white flower, also eight newe laide egges, the Whites and Yolkes beaten together, then put the said egges into the Flower, then take eight Graines of fine Milke, and stampe it in a Morter, then put halfe a pint of good Damaske water, or else rosewater into the Mulke, and mingle it together,

F 2   and

Original page from the Good Huswifes Jewel, Douce Edition, Bodleian Library, Oxford.

GLOSSARY

ALEMBIC — A close vessel for distilling

ALICOMPANE — Elecompane, enulae campanae helenij

ALOES — Any dish made with sliced meats

ARCHANGEL — Dead nettle

AVENS — Colewort or herb bonet

AYSEL — Vinegar

BALDE — Leaf

BASTARD — A sweet wine

BLANCH POWDER — Powdered spices

BOIL — Poach

BOLEARMONIACKE — A stringent earth from Armenia, a styptic or antidote

BRAY — Beat, pound, crush

BRETTE — A species of turbot

BROACH — Cooking spit

BUGLE — Bugloss

CHAFING DISH — A small portable stove

CHALDRON — Chaudron, entrails

CHEAT BREAD — A coarse bread, usually dark and of second quality

CHEWETS — Small pies

CLOD — Coarse part of an ox neck

COMODE — Mixture

CONIES — Rabbits over a year old

COPPERAS — Photosulphate of copper, iron, or zinc

COSTARDS — Apples

CREMITARIES — Turnovers

CREWS — Cruse

DRAGANT — Gum tragacanth

DRAGON — Toadflax

DRIVE — To roll out pastry

FLEA — To flay or skin

FLEAME — Phlegm

FLEATTE, FLATTE — Lard

FLOKE — Ling

FLORENTINE — Tart filled with dried fruit, spices, and chopped meat

FLOWER DE LUCE — Fleur de lys, iris pseudocorous

GALANTINE — Strong sauce

GALINGALL — Rhyzome of the ginger family

GALLIPOT, GALLY POT — Earthenware pot, glazed

GOD'S GOOD — Balm or yeast

GOLD — Gold leaves used in cooking for decoration

GOREBILL — Garfish

GROAT — Silver coin worth four pennies

GROMEL — Lithospermum

HEARNE RASE — Hair sieve

HUMBLES — Innards

ISINGLASS — Substance obtained from swim bladders of freshwater fish, used as gelatine

JULEP	Syrup
LAINE	Layer
LANGE DE BEEF	Bugloss
LASK,LASKE	Diarrhoea
LEACH, LECHE	Slice of set curds, or milk
LIGHTS	Lungs of an animal
LUTED	Stopped with clay
MANCHET	Best white bread
MARCHPANE	Ground almonds, sugar, and rose-water, now known as marz-ipan. Banqueting Stuffe
MARTINMAS BEEF	Salt beef
MAYDENS	Apples
MEAT	Food
METHRIDATUM	Candytuft, bastard methridate mustard or mustard, lepidium campestre
MILTE	Spleen
MORTISE	A dish of pounded meat, poultry, or fish
MOTHER THYME	Wild thyme, thymus serpyllum
MUGGETS	Intestines of calves or sheep
MUNDIFIED	Cleansed
MURRE	An infectious disease of cattle
NAVEN	Turnip nearest the shoulder
OCCUPTE	Make use of
OIL DE BAYE	Oil from bay berries
ORPIMENT	Arsenic trisulphide
OUIBLES	Wafers

OX WHITE	Old term for ox flank, used by butchers
PASTORNES	Pasterns
PECK	Eight quarts, or one quarter of a bushel
PELLITORY OF SPAIN	Anacyclus pyrethrum
PELLITORY OF THE WALL.	Parietaria officinalis
PENNYROYAL	Species of mint, mentha pulegeum
PHILOPENDULA	Dropwort, filipendula
POMECITRON	Fruit larger than a lemon, a hicker rind and less acid
POMPON	Large melon or pumpkin
POSNET	Small metal pot with three legs and a handle
POTTEL,POTTLE	Two quarts
PURTENANCE	Inner organs of an animal
QUAILE	Curdle
RAISINS OF THE SUN	Genuine dried large raisins, as apart from dried currants
REFECT	A portion of food
REINS	Kidneys
RESBONES	Cheesecakes
ROCHE ALAM	Rock alum
ROSASOLIS	Sundew, drosera rotundifolia
RUFFILT	Possibly a mis-spelling of refect, a portion

155

SAUNDERS	Blue colouring, azurite	TISSICK	Consumption
SEETHE	A reasonably fast boil	VAUNT	A type of fritter
SHEAL	To shell	VERJUICE	Sour juice, usually made from crab or sour apples, gooseberries, or grapes
SKIRRET	Kind of parsnip		
SMALLAGE	Parsley or celery		
SPEGALL	Spignal or spikenard		
STAMP	Grind in a mortar		
STORE	Strongly	WALME, WAUM	A period of boiling or seething
STRANGURIE	Disease of the urinary organs		
STRIKE	Stroke, rub, cut	WARDENS	Warden pears
SWEET BUTTER	Unsalted butter	WARE	Seaweed
		WHAY, WAYE	Whey
TAWNEY	Tunny	ZOYLE	Sole.

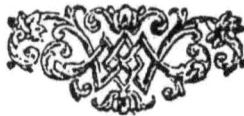

INDEX